DIABETIC FOOT CARE
HANDBOOK & JOURNAL

The Glass Foot

A Plain-English Guide for Patients Living with Diabetes

DR. JAMES WHITFIELD
Reconstructive Foot Surgeon

MELON GLOW BOOKS
Sonoma County, California
www.melonglowbooks.com

Diabetic Foot Care Handbook & Journal

The Glass Foot

Published by Melon Glow Books · Sonoma County, California

www.melonglowbooks.com

ISBN 979-8-9961392-6-2 (Paperback)

ISBN 979-8-9961392-7-9 (Hardcover)

For my patients — every one of whom taught me something.

I have spent nearly thirty years as a foot surgeon. I have operated on feet that were damaged, infected, ulcerated, and broken in every way that feet can be broken. I have sat with patients before surgery and after. I have had the conversations no one wants to have — about what happens when things are caught too late, and about what could have been done differently.

The patients I think about most are not the complicated surgical cases. They are the ones who came in with something small — a blister, a callus, a bit of redness — that had quietly been progressing for weeks because no one had told them what to look for. Because no one had explained, in plain language, what diabetes actually does to a foot, and why that changes everything about how that foot must be cared for.

That is why I wrote this book.

This is not a textbook. It is written for the person sitting at the kitchen table who has just been told they have diabetes and wants to understand what that means for their feet. Plain, direct, and honest about the stakes.

The Glass Foot is the image I always return to. Your foot contains some of the finest, most delicate blood vessels in the body. In a diabetic patient, those vessels are more fragile still. And the foot, being the farthest point from the heart, receives the least of everything the body has to offer.

But here is what I also know after thirty years: most of what goes wrong in a diabetic foot is preventable. The daily inspection. The right shoes. The early treatment of a fungal infection. The habit of shaking out your shoes every morning. These are not complicated things. They are the things that keep small problems from becoming large ones.

The journal section at the back is there for a reason. Use it. Bring it to your appointments. Let it become the record of a foot that is being watched, cared for, and protected every day.

Your feet have been carrying you all your life without asking for much in return. Now they need a little more from you. I hope this book helps you give it to them.

Dr. James Whitfield
Reconstructive Foot Surgeon · Melon Glow Books

CHAPTER ONE

What Boxers Know That Diabetic Patients Don't

The Glass Jaw and the Glass Foot

In boxing, they call it a glass jaw.

One punch in the right spot and the fight is over — no matter how strong, how fast, or how well-trained the fighter is. A glass jaw isn't something you can see from the outside. The fighter looks perfectly healthy. His corner men don't worry. The crowd doesn't notice. But underneath, there is a hidden fragility that one good hit will expose — completely and catastrophically.

Diabetes does the same thing to your feet.

It creates what I call a glass foot — a foot that looks perfectly normal, feels perfectly fine, but can be destroyed by a single small injury you never even noticed.

I spent nearly thirty years as a foot and ankle surgeon. I have stood in operating rooms and removed body parts that could have been saved had the patient come to me sooner. By the time I saw them, the damage had progressed so far that an entire team of specialists — vascular surgeons, infectious disease physicians, wound care nurses — had to be called in, and still we could not always save what should never have been lost. People who felt fine. People who thought they were careful. People who lost everything to a blister they never felt, a cut they never saw, a shoe that fit just a little too tight.

Every one of them had a glass foot. And most of them didn't know it.

HOW DIABETES CREATES THE GLASS FOOT

To understand the glass foot, you need to understand what diabetes quietly does to your feet over time — because it does it without pain, without warning, and without mercy.

It steals your nerve signals.

The medical term is peripheral neuropathy. What it means in plain English is this: the nerves in your feet stop working properly. They stop sending accurate signals to your brain. And the most important signal they stop sending is pain.

Pain is your body's alarm system. It is how you know something is wrong. When you step on a nail, pain tells you instantly. When a shoe rubs a blister, pain tells you to take it off. When a wound is getting infected, pain tells you to see a doctor.

Take away pain, and you take away every warning you have.

THE GLASS JAW vs. THE GLASS FOOT

A boxer with a glass jaw still feels the punch. He goes down, but he knows he's been hit. A diabetic patient with neuropathy may step on a tack, walk on it for three days, and never feel a thing. By the time they notice — if they notice — the wound is already infected.

It cuts off your blood supply.

Diabetes damages blood vessels throughout the body, and the vessels in the feet are among the first to suffer. Poor circulation means that when an injury occurs, the body cannot deliver the oxygen, white blood cells, and nutrients needed to heal it.

On a healthy foot, a small cut heals in days. The body rushes resources to the wound, fights off bacteria, and closes the skin quickly and cleanly.

On a glass foot, that same small cut may not heal for weeks — or ever. The blood simply cannot get there in enough quantity to do the job. Bacteria move in. The infection deepens. It reaches the bone. And at that point, the surgeon's options become very limited.

It makes you unaware of the damage.

Here is what makes the glass foot truly dangerous: the combination of these two problems. No pain to warn you. No circulation to heal you. An injury occurs. You don't feel it. You keep walking on it. The pressure and movement make it worse. The poor blood supply means it cannot heal. Days pass. Weeks pass. By the time it becomes visible — by the time the skin breaks open or the swelling appears or the odor begins — the damage has gone deep.

SURGEON'S NOTE — WHAT I HAVE SEEN

I have seen patients come into my office with wounds they had been walking on for two weeks without knowing it. I have seen bone exposed through wounds that started as blisters. I have seen injuries that, on a healthy foot, would have healed over a weekend — but on a glass foot, required a team of specialists and still ended in permanent loss. This is the glass foot. This is what diabetes does.

THE PUNCH YOU NEVER SEE COMING

A boxer with a glass jaw has one advantage: he knows about it. He trains to protect it. He keeps his guard up. He studies his opponents for the left hook that could end the fight.

Most diabetic patients never get that advantage — because nobody tells them clearly enough what they are dealing with.

They are told their blood sugar is high. They are told to watch their diet. They are given medications. But often, nobody sits them down and says: *Your feet are now made of glass. One wrong step, one ignored blister, one pair of tight shoes — and you could lose something you can never get back.*

I am telling you now.

Your feet require a different level of attention than they did before your diagnosis. Not because they look different. Not because they feel different — in fact, the loss of feeling is precisely the problem. But because the rules have changed. The margin for error that a healthy person has — the ability to ignore a small cut, to wear uncomfortable shoes for one more day, to skip checking their feet before bed — that margin is gone.

You are now handling glass. And glass requires care.

WHAT CAREFUL HANDS LOOK LIKE

When a glassblower works, he does not rush. He does not handle his work carelessly. He inspects it constantly — turning it, examining it from every angle, looking for the tiny flaw that could become a crack, the small imperfection that could spread.

That is what daily foot inspection is. It is the careful hands of someone who knows what they are working with.

THE DAILY INSPECTION — WHAT TO LOOK FOR

Every morning, before you get out of bed, look at your feet. All of them — top, bottom, between the toes, around the nails, at the heel. Use a mirror if you need to. Ask someone to help if you cannot see the bottom. What you are looking for is anything that was not there yesterday: a red spot, a small cut, a blister, a swollen area, skin that looks darker than usual, a nail that is ingrown. These are the small cracks in the glass. Caught early, many of them can be managed. Left alone, any one of them can become the punch that ends the fight.

This handbook exists so that you never get to the point where a team of specialists is required — where reconstructive foot surgery becomes the only option, where amputation enters the conversation. So let's pay attention now, before we ever get to the reconstructive stage.

A SURGEON'S PROMISE

I designed every page of this handbook from the perspective of someone who has seen what happens when the glass foot goes unprotected — and who has also seen what happens when patients take their foot care seriously.

The patients who inspect their feet every day. Who never walk barefoot. Who check their blood sugar consistently. Who bring small concerns to their doctor before they become large ones. Those patients keep their feet. They keep their independence. They keep their lives.

You are holding the tool that can make that difference. Use it every day. Take it seriously. Treat your feet the way you would treat something precious and fragile — because that is exactly what they are.

The glass foot can be protected. But only if you handle it with care.

— Dr. James Whitfield

Foot & Ankle Surgeon, Retired · Nearly 30 years of surgical practice

CHAPTER TWO

The Glass Foot

Why Diabetic Feet Demand Your Full Attention

I want you to picture something. Close your eyes for a moment and imagine that your foot — the one that carries you through every single day — is made entirely of glass. Not thick, sturdy glass, but the finest, most delicate crystal you have ever seen. The kind that rings like a bell when you tap it and shatters at the slightest wrong pressure.

Now imagine walking on that foot. Across the pavement. Across rocks. Into shoes that pinch and rub. Through summer heat and winter cold. Bearing the full weight of your body, step after step, mile after mile, year after year.

THE GLASS FOOT

Imagine your foot is made of glass. The tiny blood vessels — the capillaries and microvasculature — are as fragile as the finest crystal. In a diabetic foot, these vessels are even more delicate, and far harder to repair once damaged.

That image — the glass foot — is the one I want you to carry throughout this handbook. Because for a person living with diabetes, it is not merely a metaphor. It is closer to the truth than most patients ever realize, until it is too late.

THE INVISIBLE DAMAGE INSIDE

Deep inside the foot runs an intricate network of blood vessels. Some are large enough to see. But the ones that matter most in diabetic foot disease are the smallest ones — the capillaries and microvasculature that feed the skin, the nerves, and the tissue at the very edges of circulation. These vessels are extraordinarily fine. They are easily bruised. Easily broken. And in a diabetic patient, they are extraordinarily difficult to repair.

Here is why that matters so much: the foot is the farthest point in your body from your heart. Blood has to travel the longest distance to get there. Pressure is lower. Flow is slower. In a diabetic patient whose circulation is already compromised by years of elevated blood sugar, this becomes a serious medical vulnerability.

SURGEON'S NOTE

In nearly 30 years of foot surgery, I have seen more hospitalizations, amputations, and life-altering complications trace their origin to a small unnoticed wound on the bottom of a foot than from almost any other single cause. A blister. A callus. A pebble in a shoe. These are not small things in a diabetic patient.

THE SILENT THIEF: LOST SENSATION

One of the cruelest complications of long-term diabetes is peripheral neuropathy — the gradual loss of sensation in the feet and lower legs. Your body's normal warning system, the pain that tells you something is wrong, begins to go quiet. A cut doesn't sting the way it should. A developing ulcer on the bottom of the foot may go completely unnoticed for days.

WHEN SMALL PROBLEMS BECOME LIFE-THREATENING

A small ulcer that would heal in days in a healthy person can persist for weeks or months in a diabetic foot. As it lingers, bacteria find their way in. Infection takes hold in tissue that lacks the blood supply to fight back effectively. That local infection can deepen, reaching bone. It can spread. It can become sepsis — a life-threatening whole-body response to infection that sends patients to the hospital, and in the worst cases, to the operating room for an amputation that could have been prevented.

I do not say this to frighten you. I say it because understanding the stakes is the first step toward protecting yourself.

In the chapters ahead, we will walk through exactly how to do that — daily inspections, proper footwear, wound recognition, when to call your doctor, and the simple habits that can make an enormous difference.

CHAPTER THREE

Know Your Enemy

What Diabetes Does to the Foot

The body is a democracy, of sorts. Every organ, every limb, every system makes its demands and draws its share of the body's resources. The brain commands. The heart insists. And the feet — the feet are the quiet ones at the far end of the table, getting along on whatever is left.

> *"The feet are the poor cousins of the body — receiving less nourishment than any other part, yet soldiering on, day after day, without complaint."*

We have already discussed the distance from the heart. And as anyone knows, distance from anything can lead to neglect. Your feet know this. They soldier on regardless — through pavement and gravel, through heat and cold, bearing the full weight of everything you are. But now there is diabetes. And diabetes changes the terms of that arrangement entirely.

A THINNER DINNER PLATE

Think of it this way. Every part of your body sits down each day to a dinner plate — a share of the circulation, the oxygen, the nutrients, the healing resources your body produces. The feet have always had a smaller plate than most. They are at the end of the line.

Diabetes makes that plate thinner still.

Years of elevated blood sugar damage the walls of blood vessels — large ones and small ones alike. The fine capillaries that feed the skin and the nerves of the foot thicken and narrow. Blood flows through them more slowly, in smaller quantities, carrying less of everything the foot needs to stay healthy and repair itself.

SURGEON'S NOTE — THE WHOLE BODY IS AFFECTED

The body is compromised throughout by diabetes — the kidneys, the eyes, the cardiovascular system, the nerves. We are focusing here on the feet, but understand: what diabetes does to the foot, it is doing elsewhere too. The foot is where we see the consequences most vividly — because of where it sits at the very end of the body's supply chain.

THE ENDOCRINE SYSTEM — PLAIN ENGLISH

The endocrine system is the body's chemical messenger network — glands that produce and release hormones directly into the bloodstream. The pancreas produces insulin — the hormone that acts like a key, unlocking cells so they can absorb glucose from the blood. In Type 2 diabetes, the body either does not produce enough insulin, or the cells have become resistant to it — the locks have changed, and the old key no longer fits.

The result: glucose builds up in the bloodstream instead of entering the cells that need it. And that excess glucose quietly damages nerves, stiffens blood vessel walls, impairs the immune system, and reduces the body's capacity to heal.

THE THREE DANGERS

Neuropathy The foot loses its voice	■	Poor Circulation The dinner plate grows thinner	■	Slow Healing Wounds linger and deepen

- **Neuropathy** — nerve damage that silences the foot's alarm system. The foot can be injured and send no signal strong enough to trigger a response.
- **Poor Circulation** — damaged blood vessels mean the foot receives less blood, less oxygen, and fewer resources needed to fight infection

and heal.

• **Slow Healing** — these first two dangers combine to produce the third. A wound that would heal in days in a healthy person may take weeks or months in a diabetic foot.

Your feet have always been the quiet soldiers at the end of the line. Now they need your help — more than ever before — because the plate they are working from has never been thinner.

CHAPTER FOUR

The Daily Foot Inspection

Your Single Most Important Daily Habit

If I could give every diabetic patient one habit — just one — it would be this: look at your feet every single day. Not a glance. A real, deliberate inspection. Because the foot that cannot feel what is happening to it depends entirely on your eyes to catch what its nerves have missed.

This takes two minutes. It costs nothing. And it has prevented more amputations than any surgery I have ever performed.

WHY LOOKING REPLACES FEELING

In a healthy foot, pain is the guardian. It shouts when something is wrong. It stops you mid-step when a pebble enters your shoe. Neuropathy silences that alarm. The injury still happens — the blister, the cut, the developing ulcer — but the signal never reaches you. Your eyes must now do the job your nerves can no longer do reliably.

SURGEON'S NOTE — TWO MINUTES A DAY

I have had patients come in with wounds they had no idea existed. A nail puncture. A blister the size of a quarter. An early ulcer on the heel. Not because they were careless — but because they simply never looked. Two minutes a day changes that entirely.

THE STEP-BY-STEP ROUTINE

- **Top of the foot** — check for redness, swelling, any change in skin color, cuts, or abrasions.
- **Bottom of the foot (sole)** — use a mirror. Look at the heel, the arch, and the ball. These are the highest-pressure areas and the most

common sites for ulcers.

• **Between every toe** — spread the toes gently and look in each space. Fungal infections and skin breakdown often hide here and go undetected longest.

• **The toes and toenails** — check for ingrown nails, bruising, discoloration, or any nail that appears thickened or crumbly.

• **The heel** — feel with your fingers as well as looking. Heel cracks can be deep enough to bleed and become infected without being immediately visible.

• **Skin temperature** — run the back of your hand across both feet. One foot significantly warmer than the other is a warning sign worth investigating.

IMPORTANT — NEVER SKIP THE INSPECTION

If you cannot bend or see your feet clearly, do not skip this inspection. Ask a family member or caregiver to help. Use a long-handled mirror. Consider a podiatry appointment for professional inspection if daily self-inspection is not possible. This step is not optional.

YOUR EYES AND YOUR DOCTOR'S EYES — BOTH MATTER

Daily self-inspection is essential. But your physician's examination is something different entirely. When your doctor examines your feet, he or she is closer to them — physically, professionally, clinically — than you have ever been. The trained eye at that distance sees things a careful patient with a mirror cannot always catch: early tissue changes, subtle color shifts, the beginning of a wound that has not yet broken the surface.

SURGEON'S NOTE — YOUR EYES AND YOUR FEET

> The same fragile blood vessels causing problems in your feet are also at work in your eyes. Diabetic retinopathy — bleeding and leakage from tiny vessels in the retina — is one of the leading causes of vision loss in diabetic patients. If your vision is deteriorating — cataracts forming, sight weakening — the very eyes you rely on to inspect your feet may not be giving you a complete picture. See both your foot doctor and your eye doctor regularly. The same disease is at work in both places.

It sneaks up gradually. Do not let any of it sneak up on you. That is the lesson of this entire chapter, and of this entire book.

Your feet have been carrying you in silence for years. Now it is your turn to watch over them — and to bring in the right professional eyes to help. Two minutes every morning. Regular visits to your doctor.

CHAPTER FIVE

Footwear

The Most Underestimated Medicine

In nearly thirty years of foot surgery, I have seen many things send patients to the operating room. But I have also seen something far more preventable cause serious, lasting damage to diabetic feet: the wrong shoes. Or worse — no shoes at all.

SHAKE YOUR SHOES — EVERY SINGLE TIME

Before I say another word about footwear, I want to give you the single most important habit I teach every diabetic patient. It costs nothing. It takes three seconds. And it could save your foot.

Every morning, before you put on your shoes, pick them up and shake them out. Turn them upside down. Look inside. Every single time — not just when you think something might be in there. Because you will not always know.

SURGEON'S TIP — SHAKE YOUR SHOES FIRST

You will be surprised what has been found inside shoes before they were put on. Scorpions. Centipedes. Spiders — and their egg sacs. Bits of gravel or broken glass. A screw. A small pebble. A healthy person feels that foreign object within seconds and removes it. A diabetic patient with neuropathy may feel nothing — and walk on it all day. By the time the skin breaks, an infection is already beginning. Shake your shoes. Every time. No exceptions.

THE INVISIBLE HAZARD — TINY GLASS YOU CANNOT SEE

Think back to the last time a glass broke in your kitchen. You swept up carefully. But glass, when it shatters, does not break into pieces you can always see. The finest fragments are almost dust-like — invisible to the naked eye, light enough to drift, small enough to settle into the gap beneath a dishwasher or along a baseboard.

Then, weeks or months later, a vibration, a breeze, a door closing — and those invisible fragments migrate out onto the floor you walk on every morning. A person with normal sensation feels it immediately and demands it be removed. A diabetic patient who cannot feel it walks on that fragment all day, every step driving it slightly deeper.

A SURGEON'S REFLECTION — ANDROCLES AND THE LION

This situation always reminds me of the fable of Androcles and the Lion. Androcles encounters a lion roaring in agony in a cave. He bravely removes a large thorn buried deep in the lion's paw and cleans the wound. They part as friends. Later, Androcles is thrown into the arena to be devoured by a lion — the same one. It recognizes him, refuses to attack, and shows him only affection. The emperor, moved, frees them both. A thorn in a paw. A sliver of glass in a foot. The principle is the same: a small foreign body, left unaddressed, causes constant suffering. Removed with skill and care — it changes everything.

WHAT TO LOOK FOR IN DIABETIC-SAFE FOOTWEAR

- **Deep toe box** — enough room for all five toes to lie flat without compression.
- **Cushioned sole** — thick enough to absorb impact and protect from hard surfaces.
- **Smooth interior lining** — no prominent seams or rough stitching against the skin.
- **Adjustable closure** — laces or velcro allow you to customize fit as swelling changes through the day.

- **Breathable material** — moisture trapped inside a shoe invites fungal infection.
- **Proper length** — half an inch of space between the longest toe and the end of the shoe.

IMPORTANT — DO NOT 'BREAK IN' SHOES

Never buy shoes that feel tight and expect them to 'break in.' A diabetic foot cannot afford that process. Buy shoes that fit correctly from day one.

NEVER GO BAREFOOT — THE SURGEON'S FIRM RULE

Never walk barefoot. Not in your house. Not on the beach. Not on the grass. Not from the bed to the bathroom at 2 in the morning. I have treated patients who stepped on a staple in their own living room and did not feel it. I have treated patients who burned the soles of their feet on hot pavement at the beach and did not realize it until they saw the blisters.

Keep a pair of clean, well-fitting slippers next to your bed. Put them on before your feet touch the floor. This is not excessive caution. This is simply understanding what your foot can and cannot feel — and protecting it accordingly.

The right shoes, the right socks, the habit of shaking them out every morning, and never letting bare skin touch an unprotected floor — these carry enormous protective power for a diabetic foot.

CHAPTER SIX

Skin & Nail Care

The Details That Save Lives

We have already talked at length about the poor circulation that defines the diabetic foot — the fine, fragile vessels, the slow healing, the daily trauma of simply walking through life. Given everything we know about how the diabetic foot functions — warm, poorly circulated, often damp inside a shoe for hours at a time — it should come as no surprise that this is an excellent breeding ground for fungal infection.

FUNGAL INFECTIONS — THE QUIET THREAT THAT ESCALATES FAST

Fungi thrive in warm, moist, low-circulation environments. The diabetic foot provides exactly those conditions. Left untreated, a fungal infection softens, cracks, and breaks down the skin barrier — the body's first line of defense against bacteria. Once that barrier is breached, what began as a patch of athlete's foot can progress to a skin ulceration, then to a deeper infection, with serious consequences.

Poor Circu lation	■	Warm & Moist Foot	■	Fungal Infection	■	Skin Brea kdown	■	Ulceration

This chain is entirely preventable — but only if the fungal infection is caught and treated on time. At the first sign of infection, before the skin has been compromised.

SURGEON'S TIP — RECOGNIZE FUNGAL INFECTION EARLY

Look for: skin that appears white, soggy, or peeling between the toes. Redness, scaling, or flaking on the sole or sides of the foot. Thickened, discolored, or crumbly toenails. Any persistent itching — though many diabetic patients feel none at all. If you see any of these signs, do not wait. Treat immediately or call your doctor.

MOISTURIZING — WHAT TO USE, AND WHERE NOT TO APPLY IT

Dry, cracked skin is another entry point for infection. Poor circulation means the diabetic foot often produces less natural oil, leading to dryness — particularly on the heel, which bears tremendous daily pressure.

Moisturize your feet daily after bathing, while the skin is still slightly damp. Use a fragrance-free lotion or cream — urea-based creams (10–25%) are particularly effective for thickened or very dry skin.

IMPORTANT — NEVER MOISTURIZE BETWEEN THE TOES

Do NOT apply moisturizer between the toes. Moisture trapped in those spaces promotes exactly the warm, damp environment that fungal infections need to take hold. Between the toes stays dry.

NAIL CARE — STRAIGHT ACROSS, NEVER TOO SHORT

- **Cut straight across** — never curve the corners down into the nail groove.
- **Leave a small white margin** — do not cut so short that the nail no longer extends past the skin edge.
- **Use proper nail scissors or clippers** — clean, sharp instruments only. Dull clippers tear rather than cut.
- **File sharp edges** — use an emery board to smooth any rough corners after cutting.

- **If you cannot see or reach your feet safely** — see a podiatrist regularly for nail care.

The skin is the foot's armor. In a diabetic patient, that armor is thinner, slower to repair, and surrounded by conditions that favor its enemies. Keep it intact through daily moisturizing, early treatment of fungal infections, and careful nail care.

CHAPTER SEVEN

Red Flags

When to Call Your Doctor Immediately

Everything we have discussed in this book is aimed at prevention. But prevention is not a guarantee. When wounds develop, the single most important thing a diabetic patient can do is recognize the warning signs early and act without delay.

Time is not neutral in a diabetic foot wound. Every day of delay is a day the infection has to deepen, to spread, to establish itself in tissue that cannot fight back effectively. What is treatable on Monday with antibiotics and wound care may require surgery by Friday.

THE FIRST RULE — DO NOT WAIT

If you see any of the signs listed in this chapter — do not wait. Do not watch it for a few more days. Do not assume it will resolve on its own. Call your doctor the same day. If after hours, go to urgent care. If there is fever, spreading redness, or you feel systemically unwell — go to the ER.

WARNING SIGNS NO DIABETIC PATIENT SHOULD IGNORE

- Any wound that has not begun to improve within 24–48 hours of basic home care
- Redness spreading beyond the immediate edge of a wound
- Warmth, swelling, or tenderness in or around any wound
- Any discharge from a wound — clear, cloudy, or discolored
- A wound with an odor — a serious sign of bacterial activity
- Skin that appears dark, dusky, or black around a wound
- Fever, chills, or feeling generally unwell alongside any foot wound

- Any wound on the foot that you did not notice forming

ULCERS, INFECTION, AND THE ROAD TO AMPUTATION

A diabetic foot ulcer is an open wound — a breakdown of the skin that exposes the tissue beneath. Ulcers are often painless in patients with neuropathy, which is precisely what makes them so dangerous. Left untreated, the wound deepens, bacteria colonize it, infection spreads into surrounding tissue (cellulitis), and from there can reach the bone itself (osteomyelitis). Bone infections are extremely difficult to treat and often require surgical removal of infected bone tissue.

SURGEON'S NOTE — THE ROAD TO AMPUTATION

The road to amputation is not sudden. It is a series of missed opportunities — each one small, each one manageable, if caught and treated at the right time. A blister becomes an ulcer. An ulcer becomes infected. An infection reaches bone. Bone infection leads to the operating room. Every step of that chain can be interrupted. But only if the patient acts early.

YOU ARE AT THE CENTER OF A TEAM

By now you are beginning to realize something important: the feet we have been focusing on throughout this book are part of a whole. If you are living with diabetes, you have probably already met the team of specialists that whole person requires.

- **Your internist** — the quarterback of your overall medical care, tracking the whole picture
- **Your endocrinologist** — managing your blood sugar and the underlying diabetic condition
- **Your ophthalmologist** — watching the fragile vessels of the retina for early damage

- **Your foot surgeon or podiatrist** — protecting and treating the feet
- **And in rural areas** — the good old family doctor, quietly quarterbacking the whole effort

SURGEON'S NOTE — YOUR WHOLE TEAM IS WATCHING

No single specialist sees all of you. That is why the team exists. Be a cooperative patient. Keep your appointments with all of them. Bring your journal. Tell each one what the others have said. You are not just a foot, or an eye, or a blood sugar number. You are a whole person — and your whole team knows it.

There is no small wound in a diabetic foot. There is only a wound that has been caught early — or one that has not. The chapters you have read, and the team of professionals watching over you, give you everything you need.

BONUS CHAPTER

Gout

When the Big Toe Roars

As a foot surgeon, gout is one of the most common conditions I treat — and one of the most dramatic. When gout strikes, there is no mistaking it. Patients describe it as the worst pain they have ever felt. Grown men who have survived broken bones and major surgery tell me a gout attack brought them to their knees. The bedsheet touching the toe is agony. The air in the room feels like too much.

WHAT GOUT ACTUALLY IS

Gout is a form of inflammatory arthritis caused by the buildup of uric acid in the blood. When uric acid levels climb too high, the excess crystallizes — forming tiny, needle-sharp crystals that deposit in the joints and surrounding tissue. The big toe joint is the most common target, though the ankle, heel, and knee can all be affected.

SURGEON'S NOTE — YOU WILL KNOW WHEN IT IS GOUT

Gout attacks often strike at night — waking patients from sleep with sudden, severe pain in the big toe joint. If you have never had gout, you will know immediately when you do. Either way — call your doctor. Do not wait it out.

WHY DIABETIC PATIENTS ARE AT HIGHER RISK

High blood sugar. Insulin resistance. Excess weight. A diet heavy in red meat, organ meats, shellfish, and alcohol. All of these raise uric acid levels. All of these are also primary drivers of Type 2 diabetes. The patient who arrives in my office with a gout attack very often has a blood chemistry panel that tells a much larger story.

"High blood sugar, insulin resistance, and a diet of excess leads to a blood chemistry that is, to put it mildly, outrageous — and the kidneys are the ones paying the price."

THE KIDNEYS — THE ORGAN YOU FORGOT ABOUT

Uric acid is processed and excreted by the kidneys. When the kidneys are working well, they filter uric acid efficiently. But diabetes damages the kidneys — quietly, gradually, over years of elevated blood sugar. When the kidneys are compromised, they cannot clear uric acid as effectively. Levels build up in the blood. Crystals form. Gout follows.

IMPORTANT — GOUT IS A WHOLE-BODY WARNING SIGN

Elevated uric acid in a diabetic patient is not just a gout problem. It is a signal that the kidneys may be under stress. Your internist and endocrinologist need to know about every gout attack. Blood chemistry — uric acid, creatinine, kidney function — must be monitored regularly.

A CONVERSATION WORTH HAVING

When a patient comes in with gout — especially a diabetic patient whose blood panel tells the whole story — there is a conversation that needs to happen. Not just about the toe. About everything.

THE COUNTRY DOCTOR'S CONVERSATION

The good country doctor — the family physician who knows you and your family — has a particular gift for this moment. He will look at your chart, your blood work, and you, and put it all together. And he may well say: I want someone else in the room for this conversation. A spouse. A son or daughter. Someone who will help you listen. Because what he has to tell you is important. The blood sugar. The uric acid. The kidney numbers. The weight. The direction things are heading — and where they can go if nothing changes. That is not a conversation meant to frighten you. It is a conversation meant to save you.

WHAT TO DO WHEN GOUT STRIKES

- **Call your doctor the same day** — anti-inflammatory medications work best when started early
- **Rest the foot** — keep weight off the affected joint as much as possible
- **Elevate** — raise the foot above heart level to help reduce swelling
- **Stay hydrated** — drink plenty of water to help the kidneys flush uric acid
- **Do not self-medicate with aspirin** — aspirin can actually raise uric acid levels and worsen an attack
- **Follow up on blood chemistry** — after the attack resolves, work with your team on long-term uric acid management

Gout announces itself loudly enough that even the most reluctant patient picks up the phone. Use that moment. Call your doctor. Get the full picture. Let your team put it all together for you. That is what they are there for.

How to Use This Section

The journal pages that follow are your daily record of foot health. They are designed to take no more than two to three minutes to complete — the same two minutes you are already spending on your daily inspection.

Consistency is everything. A journal filled out six days out of seven for six months is far more valuable — to you and to your doctor — than a perfect record kept for two weeks and then abandoned.

HOW TO USE EACH DAILY LOG PAGE

- **Date & Day** — fill in at the top so your record stays in order.
- **Inspection Checklist** — check each area you examined. Circle if you found something and note it in the observations box.
- **Pain or Discomfort** — even if sensation is reduced, note any unusual feelings. Rate 0–10.
- **Skin & Nail Notes** — any changes in moisture, cracking, fungal signs, or nail appearance.
- **Footwear** — note what shoes you wore today.
- **Observations** — free space for anything you noticed. A small mark. A color change. A question for your doctor.
- **Action Taken** — note if you applied cream, treated an area, or called your doctor.

BRINGING THIS JOURNAL TO YOUR APPOINTMENTS

Bring this journal to every podiatry or physician appointment. It gives your doctor a window into what has been happening between visits — far more useful than trying to remember weeks of history on the spot. Your doctor can review trends, catch patterns, and adjust your care plan accordingly.

DAILY FOOT CARE LOG — Day 1

DATE: ______________ DAY: ______________

INSPECTION CHECKLIST (circle any area where you found an issue)

Top of foot (L)	Top of foot (R)	Sole / heel (L)
Sole / heel (R)	Between toes (L)	Between toes (R)
Toenails (L)	Toenails (R)	Skin temperature

OBSERVATIONS

____

____

____

PAIN / DISCOMFORT (0 = none 10 = severe) **0 1 2 3 4 5 6 7 8 9 10**	**FOOTWEAR WORN TODAY** ______________
SKIN & NAIL NOTES ______________ ______________	**ACTION TAKEN** ______________ ______________

FUNGAL / INFECTION SIGNS:

- ■ Peeling between toes
- ■ Scaling on sole
- ■ Discolored nail
- ■ Odor present
- ■ Redness / warmth
- ■ None observed

NOTES / QUESTIONS FOR DOCTOR

____

____

____

Diabetic Foot Care Handbook & Journal · Dr. James Whitfield · Melon Glow Books

DAILY FOOT CARE LOG — Day 2

DATE: ______________ DAY: ______________

INSPECTION CHECKLIST (circle any area where you found an issue)

Top of foot (L)	Top of foot (R)	Sole / heel (L)
Sole / heel (R)	Between toes (L)	Between toes (R)
Toenails (L)	Toenails (R)	Skin temperature

OBSERVATIONS

____

____

____

PAIN / DISCOMFORT (0 = none 10 = severe) **0 1 2 3 4 5 6 7 8 9 10**	**FOOTWEAR WORN TODAY** ______________
SKIN & NAIL NOTES ______________ ______________	**ACTION TAKEN** ______________ ______________

FUNGAL / INFECTION SIGNS:

■ Peeling between toes ■ Scaling on sole ■ Discolored nail

■ Odor present ■ Redness / warmth ■ None observed

NOTES / QUESTIONS FOR DOCTOR

____

____

____

Diabetic Foot Care Handbook & Journal · Dr. James Whitfield · Melon Glow Books

DAILY FOOT CARE LOG — Day 3

DATE: ____________________ **DAY:** ______________

INSPECTION CHECKLIST (circle any area where you found an issue)

Top of foot (L)	Top of foot (R)	Sole / heel (L)
Sole / heel (R)	Between toes (L)	Between toes (R)
Toenails (L)	Toenails (R)	Skin temperature

OBSERVATIONS

____

____

____

PAIN / DISCOMFORT (0 = none 10 = severe) **0 1 2 3 4 5 6 7 8 9 10**	**FOOTWEAR WORN TODAY** ____________________
SKIN & NAIL NOTES ____________________ ____________________	**ACTION TAKEN** ____________________ ____________________

FUNGAL / INFECTION SIGNS:

- ■ Peeling between toes
- ■ Scaling on sole
- ■ Discolored nail
- ■ Odor present
- ■ Redness / warmth
- ■ None observed

NOTES / QUESTIONS FOR DOCTOR

____

____

____

Diabetic Foot Care Handbook & Journal · Dr. James Whitfield · Melon Glow Books

DAILY FOOT CARE LOG Day 4

DATE: ______________________ **DAY:** ________________

INSPECTION CHECKLIST (circle any area where you found an issue)

Top of foot (L)	Top of foot (R)	Sole / heel (L)
Sole / heel (R)	Between toes (L)	Between toes (R)
Toenails (L)	Toenails (R)	Skin temperature

OBSERVATIONS

____

____

____

PAIN / DISCOMFORT (0 = none 10 = severe) **0 1 2 3 4 5 6 7 8 9 10**	**FOOTWEAR WORN TODAY** ____________________
SKIN & NAIL NOTES ____________________ ____________________	**ACTION TAKEN** ____________________ ____________________

FUNGAL / INFECTION SIGNS:

■ Peeling between toes ■ Scaling on sole ■ Discolored nail

■ Odor present ■ Redness / warmth ■ None observed

NOTES / QUESTIONS FOR DOCTOR

____

____

____

Diabetic Foot Care Handbook & Journal · Dr. James Whitfield · Melon Glow Books

DAILY FOOT CARE LOG — Day 5

DATE: ____________________ **DAY:** ______________

INSPECTION CHECKLIST (circle any area where you found an issue)

Top of foot (L)	Top of foot (R)	Sole / heel (L)
Sole / heel (R)	Between toes (L)	Between toes (R)
Toenails (L)	Toenails (R)	Skin temperature

OBSERVATIONS

PAIN / DISCOMFORT (0 = none 10 = severe)

0 1 2 3 4 5 6 7 8 9 10

FOOTWEAR WORN TODAY

SKIN & NAIL NOTES

ACTION TAKEN

FUNGAL / INFECTION SIGNS:

- ■ Peeling between toes
- ■ Scaling on sole
- ■ Discolored nail
- ■ Odor present
- ■ Redness / warmth
- ■ None observed

NOTES / QUESTIONS FOR DOCTOR

Diabetic Foot Care Handbook & Journal · Dr. James Whitfield · Melon Glow Books

DAILY FOOT CARE LOG — Day 6

DATE: ______________________ **DAY:** ________________

INSPECTION CHECKLIST (circle any area where you found an issue)

Top of foot (L)	Top of foot (R)	Sole / heel (L)
Sole / heel (R)	Between toes (L)	Between toes (R)
Toenails (L)	Toenails (R)	Skin temperature

OBSERVATIONS

____

____

____

PAIN / DISCOMFORT (0 = none 10 = severe) **0 1 2 3 4 5 6 7 8 9 10**	**FOOTWEAR WORN TODAY** ______________________
SKIN & NAIL NOTES ______________________ ______________________	**ACTION TAKEN** ______________________ ______________________

FUNGAL / INFECTION SIGNS:

- ■ Peeling between toes
- ■ Scaling on sole
- ■ Discolored nail
- ■ Odor present
- ■ Redness / warmth
- ■ None observed

NOTES / QUESTIONS FOR DOCTOR

____

____

____

Diabetic Foot Care Handbook & Journal · Dr. James Whitfield · Melon Glow Books

DAILY FOOT CARE LOG Day 7

DATE: ____________________ **DAY:** ______________

INSPECTION CHECKLIST (circle any area where you found an issue)

Top of foot (L)	Top of foot (R)	Sole / heel (L)
Sole / heel (R)	Between toes (L)	Between toes (R)
Toenails (L)	Toenails (R)	Skin temperature

OBSERVATIONS

____

____

____

PAIN / DISCOMFORT (0 = none 10 = severe) **0 1 2 3 4 5 6 7 8 9 10**	**FOOTWEAR WORN TODAY** ______________________
SKIN & NAIL NOTES ______________________ ______________________	**ACTION TAKEN** ______________________ ______________________

FUNGAL / INFECTION SIGNS:

- ■ Peeling between toes
- ■ Scaling on sole
- ■ Discolored nail
- ■ Odor present
- ■ Redness / warmth
- ■ None observed

NOTES / QUESTIONS FOR DOCTOR

____

____

____

Diabetic Foot Care Handbook & Journal · Dr. James Whitfield · Melon Glow Books

WEEKLY SUMMARY & DOCTOR'S NOTES

WEEK OF: ______________________________

OVERALL ASSESSMENT THIS WEEK:

- ■ No issues — feet in good condition
- ■ Minor issue identified and treated
- ■ Issue present — monitoring closely
- ■ Called / saw doctor this week

ISSUES OR CONCERNS THIS WEEK:

TREATMENTS OR ACTIONS TAKEN:

QUESTIONS TO ASK MY DOCTOR AT NEXT VISIT:

DOCTOR'S NOTES / APPOINTMENT SUMMARY:

Diabetic Foot Care Handbook & Journal · Dr. James Whitfield · Melon Glow Books

WEEKLY SUMMARY & DOCTOR'S NOTES

WEEK OF: ______________________________

OVERALL ASSESSMENT THIS WEEK:

- ■ No issues — feet in good condition
- ■ Minor issue identified and treated
- ■ Issue present — monitoring closely
- ■ Called / saw doctor this week

ISSUES OR CONCERNS THIS WEEK:

TREATMENTS OR ACTIONS TAKEN:

QUESTIONS TO ASK MY DOCTOR AT NEXT VISIT:

DOCTOR'S NOTES / APPOINTMENT SUMMARY:

Diabetic Foot Care Handbook & Journal · Dr. James Whitfield · Melon Glow Books

MEDICATION LOG

A Complete Record for Your Entire Care Team

Your medications are a critical part of managing diabetes and protecting your feet. This log is designed to be brought to every appointment so your entire care team can see at a glance what you are taking, at what dose, and for how long. Never stop or change a medication without consulting your physician. Note any side effects you observe, particularly any that affect your feet or legs.

MEDICATION LOG

List all medications — prescription, over-the-counter, and supplements. Bring this log to every appointment.

Medication Name	Dose	Frequency	Prescribing Doctor	Start Date	Notes / Side Effects
1					
2					
3					
4					
5					
6					
7					
8					
9					
10					
11					
12					
13					
14					

KNOWN ALLERGIES / DRUG REACTIONS:

MEDICATION LOG

List all medications — prescription, over-the-counter, and supplements. Bring this log to every appointment.

Medication Name	Dose	Frequency	Prescribing Doctor	Start Date	Notes / Side Effects
15					
16					
17					
18					
19					
20					
21					
22					
23					
24					
25					
26					
27					
28					

KNOWN ALLERGIES / DRUG REACTIONS:

BLOOD SUGAR LOG

Daily Glucose Tracking — Fasting & Post-Meal

Blood sugar management is the foundation of diabetic foot protection. Elevated glucose damages the blood vessels and nerves that your feet depend on. This log tracks your fasting reading — taken before eating in the morning — and your post-meal reading, taken two hours after a meal. Your target ranges will be set by your physician, but in general: fasting below 130 mg/dL and post-meal below 180 mg/dL are commonly recommended starting points. Consistent logging over 60 days gives your doctor a far clearer picture than a single office reading ever can.

BLOOD SUGAR LOG

TARGET RANGES (confirm with doctor): Fasting: under 130 mg/dL | Post-Meal (2 hrs): under 180 mg/dL | Mark

Day	Date	Fasting (mg/dL)	Post-Meal (mg/dL)	Time Taken	Notes / How Feeling
1					
2					
3					
4					
5					
6					
7					
8					
9					
10					
11					
12					
13					
14					
15					

BLOOD SUGAR LOG

TARGET RANGES (confirm with doctor): Fasting: under 130 mg/dL | Post-Meal (2 hrs): under 180 mg/dL |

Day	Date	Fasting (mg/dL)	Post-Meal (mg/dL)	Time Taken	Notes / How Feeling
16					
17					
18					
19					
20					
21					
22					
23					
24					
25					
26					
27					
28					
29					
30					

BLOOD SUGAR LOG

TARGET RANGES (confirm with doctor): Fasting: under 130 mg/dL | Post-Meal (2 hrs): under 180 mg/dL | Mark

Day	Date	Fasting (mg/dL)	Post-Meal (mg/dL)	Time Taken	Notes / How Feeling
31					
32					
33					
34					
35					
36					
37					
38					
39					
40					
41					
42					
43					
44					
45					

BLOOD SUGAR LOG

TARGET RANGES (confirm with doctor): Fasting: under 130 mg/dL | Post-Meal (2 hrs): under 180 mg/dL |

Day	Date	Fasting (mg/dL)	Post-Meal (mg/dL)	Time Taken	Notes / How Feeling
46					
47					
48					
49					
50					
51					
52					
53					
54					
55					
56					
57					
58					
59					
60					

WOUND & INCIDENT LOG

A Permanent Record of Every Skin Event

In a diabetic foot, there is no such thing as a wound too small to document. This log creates a permanent record of every cut, blister, abrasion, redness, or skin change you notice — when it appeared, where it was located, what you did, and how it resolved. Over time, this record reveals patterns your doctor can use to identify problems before they become serious. When in doubt, document it.

WOUND & INCIDENT LOG

Document every skin change, cut, blister, redness, or wound — no matter how minor it appears.

INCIDENT #1

Date noticed: **Left / Right foot:**

Location on foot:

Description:

Action taken: **Outcome:**

Called doctor? ■ **Yes** ■ **No** **Instructions:**

INCIDENT #2

Date noticed: **Left / Right foot:**

Location on foot:

Description:

Action taken: **Outcome:**

Called doctor? ■ **Yes** ■ **No** **Instructions:**

INCIDENT #3

Date noticed: **Left / Right foot:**

Location on foot:

Description:

Action taken: **Outcome:**

Called doctor? ■ **Yes** ■ **No** **Instructions:**

INCIDENT #4

Date noticed: **Left / Right foot:**

Location on foot:

Description:

Action taken: **Outcome:**

Called doctor? ■ **Yes** ■ **No** **Instructions:**

WOUND & INCIDENT LOG

Document every skin change, cut, blister, redness, or wound — no matter how minor it appears.

INCIDENT #5

Date noticed: **Left / Right foot:**

Location on foot:

Description:

Action taken: **Outcome:**

Called doctor? ■ **Yes** ■ **No** **Instructions:**

INCIDENT #6

Date noticed: **Left / Right foot:**

Location on foot:

Description:

Action taken: **Outcome:**

Called doctor? ■ **Yes** ■ **No** **Instructions:**

INCIDENT #7

Date noticed: **Left / Right foot:**

Location on foot:

Description:

Action taken: **Outcome:**

Called doctor? ■ **Yes** ■ **No** **Instructions:**

INCIDENT #8

Date noticed: **Left / Right foot:**

Location on foot:

Description:

Action taken: **Outcome:**

Called doctor? ■ **Yes** ■ **No** **Instructions:**

MY CARE TEAM

Every Specialist. Every Number. In One Place.

Bring this page to every appointment. When one specialist asks who else you are seeing, you will have the answer at your fingertips.

Primary Care / Internist

The quarterback of your overall medical care

Name: ______________________ Phone: ______________________

Endocrinologist

Manages your diabetes, blood sugar, and insulin

Name: ______________________ Phone: ______________________

Foot Surgeon / Podiatrist

Protects and treats your feet

Name: ______________________ Phone: ______________________

Ophthalmologist / Eye Doctor

Monitors diabetic changes in the retina

Name: ______________________ Phone: ______________________

Cardiologist

Monitors cardiovascular health

Name: ______________________ Phone: ______________________

Vascular Surgeon

Evaluates blood flow to the legs and feet

Name: ______________________ Phone: ______________________

Wound Care Specialist

Manages chronic or complex wounds

Name: ______________________ Phone: ______________________

Pharmacist

Reviews medications and interactions

Name: ______________________ Phone: ______________________

UPCOMING APPOINTMENTS

Write your questions down before each appointment — you will remember more and your doctor will appreciate it.

1
Date & Time: **Doctor:**
Purpose:
Questions:

2
Date & Time: **Doctor:**
Purpose:
Questions:

3
Date & Time: **Doctor:**
Purpose:
Questions:

4
Date & Time: **Doctor:**
Purpose:
Questions:

5
Date & Time: **Doctor:**
Purpose:
Questions:

6
Date & Time: **Doctor:**
Purpose:
Questions:

7
Date & Time: **Doctor:**
Purpose:
Questions:

APPOINTMENT SUMMARY

Date of appointment:

Doctor / Specialist seen:

Location / Clinic:

Reason for visit:

WHAT THE DOCTOR FOUND

CHANGES TO MEDICATIONS OR TREATMENT

INSTRUCTIONS GIVEN

FOLLOW-UP REQUIRED

MY NOTES & QUESTIONS FOR NEXT TIME

APPOINTMENT SUMMARY

Date of appointment:

Doctor / Specialist seen:

Location / Clinic:

Reason for visit:

WHAT THE DOCTOR FOUND

CHANGES TO MEDICATIONS OR TREATMENT

INSTRUCTIONS GIVEN

FOLLOW-UP REQUIRED

MY NOTES & QUESTIONS FOR NEXT TIME

UNDERSTANDING YOUR A1C

The Single Most Important Number in Diabetic Foot Health

A plain-English explanation from Dr. James Whitfield

If you have diabetes, you have probably had your A1C tested. But many patients leave the office without a clear understanding of what that number actually means — and why it matters so profoundly for the health of their feet.

WHAT THE A1C MEASURES

The A1C test measures your average blood sugar level over the past two to three months — not just what it was this morning, but the cumulative picture. It measures how much glucose has attached to the hemoglobin in your red blood cells. A higher A1C means higher average blood sugar over that period.

A1C Level	What It Means	Avg Blood Sugar
Below 5.7%	Normal	Below 117 mg/dL
5.7% – 6.4%	Pre-diabetes	117–137 mg/dL
6.5% and above	Diabetes	137+ mg/dL
Below 7.0%	Well-managed (target)	Below 154 mg/dL
7.0% – 8.0%	Moderate — room to improve	154–183 mg/dL
Above 8.0%	Elevated risk — feet in danger	Above 183 mg/dL

WHY THIS MATTERS FOR YOUR FEET: Every point your A1C rises above 7.0% represents meaningful additional damage to the blood vessels and nerves that protect your feet. The goal of this journal is to give you and your doctor the tools to keep that number where it needs to be.

Ask your doctor what your personal A1C target is, and write it here: ____________ Ask how often it should be tested: ____________

SHOE & INSOLE RECORD

Track What You Wear — Your Feet Depend On It

The shoes you wear are the single most controllable risk factor in diabetic foot protection. This record helps you track each pair — when you bought them, any problems they caused, and when they need replacing. A good diabetic shoe typically needs replacement every 6–12 months. Never wear a shoe that caused a blister or skin irritation without having it assessed.

SHOE / INSOLE #1

Brand / Model: **Size:** **Date purchased:**

Type: ■ **Everyday** ■ **Diabetic/Therapeutic** ■ **Athletic** ■ **Dress** ■ **Slipper** ■ **Insole only**

Fit notes / problems: ■ **In use** ■ **Retired**

SHOE / INSOLE #2

Brand / Model: **Size:** **Date purchased:**

Type: ■ **Everyday** ■ **Diabetic/Therapeutic** ■ **Athletic** ■ **Dress** ■ **Slipper** ■ **Insole only**

Fit notes / problems: ■ **In use** ■ **Retired**

SHOE / INSOLE #3

Brand / Model: **Size:** **Date purchased:**

Type: ■ **Everyday** ■ **Diabetic/Therapeutic** ■ **Athletic** ■ **Dress** ■ **Slipper** ■ **Insole only**

Fit notes / problems: ■ **In use** ■ **Retired**

SHOE / INSOLE #4

Brand / Model: **Size:** **Date purchased:**

Type: ■ **Everyday** ■ **Diabetic/Therapeutic** ■ **Athletic** ■ **Dress** ■ **Slipper** ■ **Insole only**

Fit notes / problems: ■ **In use** ■ **Retired**

SHOE / INSOLE #5

Brand / Model: **Size:** **Date purchased:**

Type: ■ **Everyday** ■ **Diabetic/Therapeutic** ■ **Athletic** ■ **Dress** ■ **Slipper** ■ **Insole only**

Fit notes / problems: ■ **In use** ■ **Retired**

SHOE / INSOLE #6

Brand / Model: **Size:** **Date purchased:**

Type: ■ **Everyday** ■ **Diabetic/Therapeutic** ■ **Athletic** ■ **Dress** ■ **Slipper** ■ **Insole only**

Fit notes / problems: ■ **In use** ■ **Retired**

QUICK REFERENCE

Daily Diabetic Foot Care At a Glance

EVERY MORNING

✓ Shake out both shoes and look inside before putting them on

✓ Put on clean, seamless, moisture-wicking socks

✓ Slippers first — never bare feet on the floor

DAILY FOOT INSPECTION

✓ Top of both feet — color, swelling, any new marks

✓ Bottom (sole) — use a mirror; check heel, arch, ball

✓ Between every toe — spread and look carefully

✓ Toenails — discoloration, thickness, ingrown edges

✓ Temperature — one warmer foot is a warning sign

SKIN & NAIL CARE

✓ Moisturize daily after bathing — NOT between the toes

✓ Cut toenails straight across, never too short

✓ Treat any fungal signs immediately — do not wait

✓ No razor blades or chemical corn removers

CALL YOUR DOCTOR TODAY IF:

• Any wound not improving within 24–48 hours • Redness or swelling spreading outward from a wound • Any discharge, odor, or darkening of tissue • Fever or feeling unwell alongside any foot wound • Any wound you did not feel forming

THE SURGEON'S FIRM RULES

• Never go barefoot — not even across the room • Never buy tight shoes expecting to break them in • Never ignore a small wound — there is no small wound here • Never delay calling your doctor when a red flag appears

---

Dr. James Whitfield

Reconstructive Foot Surgeon

Dr. James Whitfield is a reconstructive foot surgeon with nearly thirty years of clinical practice, licensed across multiple states. Over the course of his career he has treated thousands of patients suffering from conditions ranging from acute foot injuries to the complex, chronic complications of diabetic foot disease.

His approach to patient care has always been grounded in plain-language education — the belief that patients who understand what is happening in their bodies make better decisions and achieve better outcomes. It is this philosophy that led him to write the Diabetic Foot Care Handbook & Journal.

His clinical experience encompasses reconstructive foot surgery, diabetic wound care, limb salvage, and the surgical management of foot and ankle disorders. He has seen firsthand the difference that early education and daily vigilance make in the lives of diabetic patients — and the devastating consequences when that knowledge is absent.

Dr. Whitfield publishes under the Melon Glow Books imprint, an independent publishing house dedicated to bringing expert medical knowledge to everyday readers in accessible, beautifully crafted books.

Melon Glow Books · Sonoma County, California

ALSO FROM DR. JAMES WHITFIELD

If you have read this far, you already know something important: diabetes does not affect the foot in isolation. It changes the entire environment in which your feet must live and function.

And there is another category of foot conditions that diabetic patients face at higher rates, with more serious consequences — the mechanical and inflammatory conditions that create exactly the kind of pressure, friction, and tissue stress that a diabetic foot can least afford.

Plantar fasciitis. Bone spurs. Arthritis. Gout. The next book in this series was written for you.

COMING NEXT FROM MELON GLOW BOOKS

Plantar Fasciitis, Bone Spurs, Arthritis and Gout

Oh My!

A Plain English Guide for Diabetic Patients

Dr. James Whitfield

In the same plain-English style as this handbook, Dr. Whitfield walks you through each of these conditions — what causes them, what they feel like, and what can be done about them. With special attention throughout to the diabetic patient.

Watch for it at melonglowbooks.com and wherever books are sold.

www.melonglowbooks.com · Support@melonglowbooks.com

www.ingramcontent.com/pod-product-compliance
Lightning Source LLC
LaVergne TN
LVHW011816200926
848484LV00005B/1218

CULTURE OF TRUST

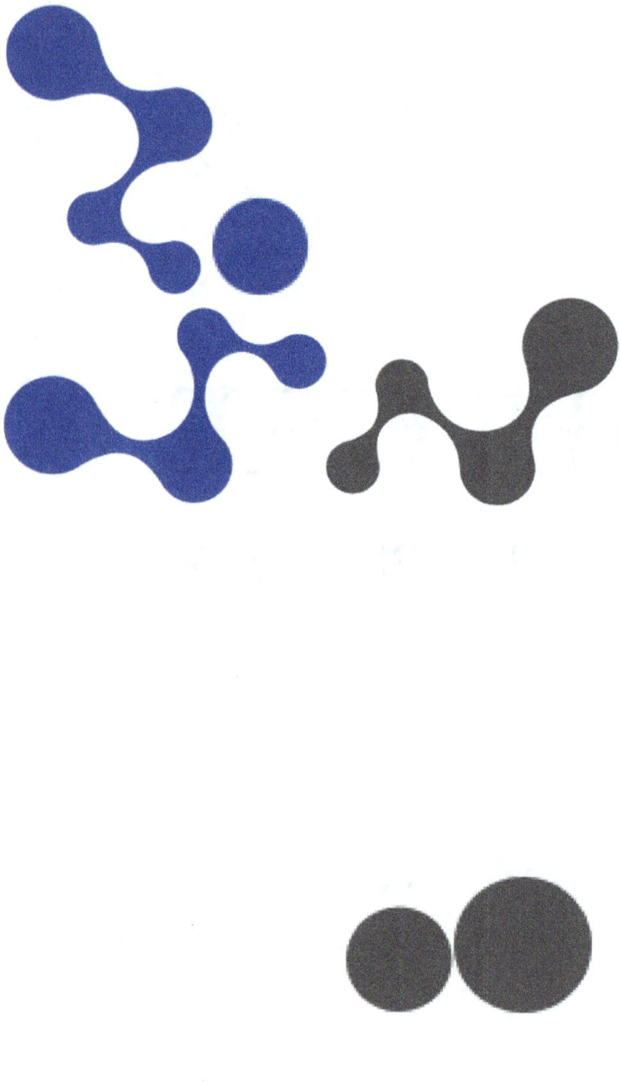

LUIZ FRANÇA

CULTURE OF TRUST

The art of engagement for strong teams that generate results

ISBN: 979-8-9943815-2-6
Imprint: EssenceBiz

Cover design by: Jamile Buck
Illustrative Image from: @EyeEm / Freepik

Printed in the United States of America

THANKS!

To Ilma, Luana, Malu, Teca, and Jacinto—thank you for filling my life with the most extraordinary energy and vital vibrations, propelling me forward with hope and purpose. Your unwavering support and encouragement have been the light that guided me through this journey.

I also dedicate this work to all the marvelous people who have shared the path of life with me, enriching my days with their wisdom, kindness, and authenticity. Through our interactions, you have taught me invaluable lessons and inspired me to grow into a better version of myself. Your presence has been unforgettable, and your friendship a gift I will forever cherish.

This book is for you all, with deep gratitude and immense affection.

Contents

PREFACE

Those who live in the corporate world know all too well that the main topics of discussion are metrics, goals, achievements, growth, evolution, records, and other buzzwords that continually echo in our minds. We are accustomed to the idea of "sweating it out" and spending sleepless nights, all for the sake of one word that motivates but also haunts many people: results. However, today, everything is changing. Yes, all of those terms remain important for the survival and growth of businesses. I myself use them frequently in my daily life. But we are now facing a reality that has shown us something different: **results for the sake of results are no longer enough.**

In fact, let me put it more clearly: results for the sake of results are what will ultimately sink your company!

We live in a reality far removed from the one where Chaplin tightened screws on a factory conveyor belt—or so we think—but even now, a significant problem persists in corporations. Only recently has this issue begun to receive the attention it demands in today's economy: the relationship between team engagement and productivity.

Developing a culture that not only promotes the well-being of employees but also gives meaning to what they do every day has become essential. It directly impacts the numbers we want to see at the end of the quarter. Moreover, in my opinion, it is a principle that every manager should uphold in relation to those who work hard to advance the company.

The world is constantly evolving, and so should your business!

One certainty I carry is that I'm never alone in this endeavor—a sentiment I know is common among leaders in the business world. This is because I have a small but exceptional team that believes in the company's mission and truly gives their all to achieve our objectives.

However, I didn't learn to manage teams overnight, especially since, at the beginning of my career, the relationships between different hierarchical levels in companies were very different from what they are today. Much has changed, and much is still changing, which is why we need someone like Luiz França to illuminate the path ahead.

Can you feel the weight of the issue that will be addressed in this deeply well-structured book by Luiz França? I am not here to talk to you about your illustrious career or your outstanding results. Instead, I am here to show you how the pages ahead can make a difference in your rise within the market where you work.

At the beginning of 2020, for instance, we witnessed the emergence of a new business landscape in which many companies struggled, and all had to adapt. Initially, the need arose to implement remote work, which pleased many employees. A study by Sodexo Research[1] showed that at first, 70% of people praised the practice of remote work. However, just three months into this model, the satisfaction rate dropped to 45%. This occurred because companies, in their rush to adapt, lost their way in a chaotic environment where everyone was just trying to survive.

I also want to draw your attention to another wave that arrived in mid-2020—quieter but for which we were equally unprepared: the so-called Generation Z. These new professionals, freshly graduated from universities worldwide, do not work in the same way as previous generations. Their ambitions are different, their behavior is distinct, and their relationship between work and personal life is entirely new. Who was ready to face these young pioneers and entrepreneurs who reject rigid schedules and environments that fail to promote motivation?

I know I wasn't ready for either wave, but I sought to learn and grow from them. And I'm here to show you that it was possible to adapt effectively, even under so much pressure.

It's pointless to recognize a need but ignore the changes required along the way. Today, you hold in your hands a book crafted with deep dedication to offer a simpler, less painful, and faster path for your company to effectively build more engaged teams and achieve all desired objectives.

Within these pages, you'll find a helping hand, extended and ready to guide you through this process. And here's my final tip: dive deep into this work, and you'll emerge with a new path to the success of your business.

Accept the challenge, and enjoy the read!

Ricardo Shinyashiki
Founder of GenteLab

INTRODUCTION

REDEFINING THE ROLE OF ORGANIZATIONS

It was the second half of 2010 when I first envisioned Culture of Trust. At that time, I brought with me an extensive professional background, having worked in several multinational and large national companies. My journey already spanned more than two decades of navigating challenges in people management processes. Yet, I couldn't grasp why it was so difficult to uncover the formula for engagement and happiness at work. I longed for something practical, something that transcended operational manuals. I dreamed of discovering and sharing the essence of it all.

By then, I had plenty of stories to tell—about what worked and what didn't. Yet, there was still a sense of discomfort within me. I felt that my experiences would be more meaningful if I had gone through a complete cycle, putting into practice new successes and failures to share with the world. I already had the frustrations and the aspirations. I carried a genuine desire to improve work environments and a deep belief that the business world serves as a primary engine for societal evolution and the transformation of humanity.

When I was invited to take on the role of managing people at a multinational company with an industrial plant in northeastern Brazil, I faced a unique challenge. The company required a cultural transformation and the establishment of a corporate identity for its workforce, who still associated the organization with its pre-acquisition brand. Business results were far below the expectations of its new shareholders.

I accepted this challenge in the last quarter of 2010, driven by the relentless pursuit to consolidate every people management practice I had learned. I resolved to revisit every concept with fresh experiences, extracting the essence of transformation in a clear and applicable way. My goal was to share it with as many people as possible, using every available tool to broaden access.

We started with an engagement rate of just 16%, and I thought nothing could be harder than what lay ahead. Every conventional indicator pointed to the worst possible outcome. Our management model faced criticism from institutions and individuals alike. Most troubling, we lacked the trust of our own people. The chaos we were in made any talk of change seem like a facade, a lie, or just a ploy to boost profitability. Ironically, there was no profitability—our results were public, as the company was a corporation, and the uncertainty about the future was overwhelming.

We faced difficult times, and giving up seemed like an easy option. We could have accepted poor performance as inevitable. Instead, I chose to draw upon our history of learning and build a real organization through actions designed to foster engagement. This was no theoretical exercise; it was real-world experience, complete with all the risks of managing a large-scale business.

Today, I can share every practical action I implemented to develop leaders and manage people effectively. These strategies formed a clear and actionable sequence, delivering proven results. Our journey took us from 16% engagement to becoming recognized as the best company to work for in Brazil, with the highest Happiness at Work Index (IFT).

Initially, everything seemed murky. Our priority was to understand which businesses were succeeding with high profitability and which were struggling with low performance. We needed to pinpoint what differentiated them in the market and study the behavior of companies globally.

One common factor among high-reputation, high-performance companies was their consistent ranking among the best workplaces in their countries. Their success wasn't sporadic or the result of temporary actions—it was rooted in sustained excellence.

Another critical insight was that high-performing companies were increasingly reflecting on their purpose in the world. They evaluated their performance beyond financial results. We found that the highest levels of profitability were linked to the solutions these organizations provided to the world, transforming their markets and environments.

At the core of this transformation process was leadership. It was essential to understand the practices of these leaders—their styles, their guiding purposes, and how they developed talent and cultivated a generation of capable individuals, not just for work but for life.

Through this journey of people development, we gained a deeper understanding of the power of purpose and its role in shaping organizational culture. We identified the pillars of excellent management and what sets apart those who achieve remarkable success. Understanding the tools that make a difference in professional performance was also vital.

I'm talking about administrative tools that break free from current models and disrupt cycles of social conformity in business management. These tools helped us reposition ourselves, but nothing was as effective as the coherence and consistency of our beliefs and actions—always placing people at the center of every decision. We strengthened the conviction that people are the sole reason businesses exist.

Without people, there are no ventures. The energy people dedicate to their projects, bringing the best of their potential, enhances the experiences that impact another critical group: the customers.

The art of engagement involves powerful tools to delight people at every level of business. Above all, it requires us to challenge our beliefs about management models and rethink our practices, ensuring that everything we do has a clear purpose.

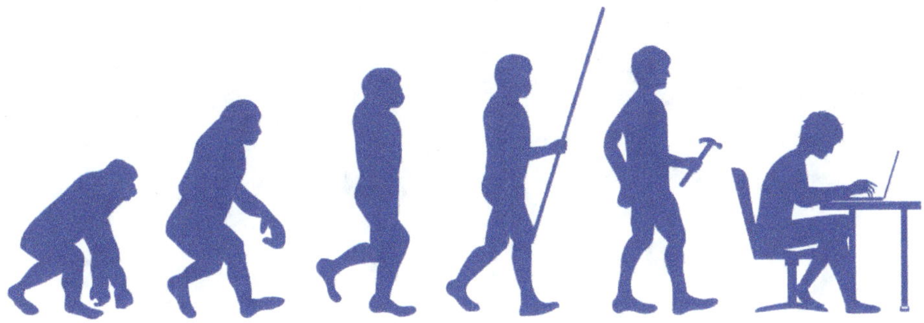

TO EVOLVE AND TO SERVE will be the essence of everything I present in this book. Together, we will learn how to make leadership a force that radiates energy and transforms lives. By doing so, we can help people live their best every day, constantly evolving and serving others. This redefines work's role in our lives and accelerates the changes businesses need, creating cycles of prosperity for the entire ecosystem.

**Engagement will be
the driving force that
empowers people to take pride
in what they do,
become true brand ambassadors,
and live their best selves every day
in an environment that fosters growth.
It will elevate work
and humanity to
a new dimension,
generating happiness
and prosperity for all.**

CHAPTER 1

TALKING IS EASY, SOLVING MY REALITY IS THE CHALLENGE

When the starting point goes beyond the challenges faced by others

When I engage in conversations with business owners, executives, leaders, and professionals, it's clear that corporate environments often share a set of deep, common pains. These challenges obscure our vision of the future and make it difficult to determine the immediate steps required to achieve meaningful cultural transformation.

The situations we navigate and the obstacles we face are always marked by unique complexities that can be hard to manage. That's why I believe it's important to share the recurring arguments I hear across various business contexts, allowing us to better understand the struggles that afflict so many of us.

Realizing that I wasn't alone in facing these challenges was a turning point. It became clear that many others were seeking solutions to the same problems I was experiencing. It's equally essential to recognize that when we transform our challenges into achievements, we create opportunities to share those breakthroughs with others. This reinforces the idea that we are deeply social beings and that our struggles, no matter how personal they feel, are often mirrored by others.

The need to overcome management challenges exists at every level and in every group. These challenges directly impact the social fabric, both through the influence organizations exert on their environments and the influence they receive in return.

In countless discussions about the transformations, I've experienced and led during my entrepreneurial journey, one theme emerges time and again: **people often believe their challenges are uniquely difficult, perhaps even insurmountable.**

When I took the first steps in designing this project, it was impossible to know whether it would succeed in creating real organizational transformation. We started with the need to manage chaotic contexts that, to us, seemed unparalleled. Yet as I describe these challenges here, you—whether a manager, executive, entrepreneur, or business owner—may recognize some of the same adversities surrounding your strategy. These situations demand immense creativity, resilience, and vision to navigate effectively.

Challenges for Senior Leadership

One of the first and most relentless challenges keeping us awake at night is financial management—balancing revenue with commitments. In chaotic situations, planning to stabilize income and expenses often feels like an impossible puzzle. We look inward and feel as though no one else cares about the situation. Meanwhile, in the market, clients negotiate longer payment terms to improve their own cash flow, putting additional strain on us. In the scramble for survival, it can feel as though there's no way out.

But it doesn't stop there. Creditors sense our vulnerability and push for renegotiated terms—suddenly, the promises of "eternal partnerships" seem like empty words. If that weren't enough, suppliers demand contract adjustments, and it seems as though competitors are being prioritized with favorable deals. Reading the news, you see your competitors expanding their markets and allocating capital to ambitious growth plans, compounding the frustration.

Internally, the situation often feels even more dire. Departments are at odds with one another, locked in blame games. Employees express dissatisfaction, feeling undervalued and under-resourced. You observe a lack of commitment and performance, and projects either stall or never get off the ground. Employees are quick to accept external offers, leaving your company for seemingly greener and more trustable places.

As if this weren't enough, internal challenges often spill over into external scrutiny. Complaints and leaks from within the organization—whether from employees or unions—trigger investigations by labor regulators, adding another layer of pressure. Prosecutors and auditors arrive, scrutinizing every detail of your management practices.

In these moments, it's easy to feel as though the world is conspiring against you. It can seem like there are individuals who dedicate themselves entirely to causing your organization to fail.

Executives and entrepreneurs often express frustration that despite investing heavily in their business strategies, there's a lack of understanding and commitment from their teams. Even after significant investments in communication—using simple language, visuals, and diverse methods to convey the message—the results are underwhelming.

Compounding this issue are unstable external variables that disrupt business plans. Legislative changes, unreliable regulatory frameworks, and costly adaptations create roadblocks that hinder decision-making and execution.

Balancing the four critical pillars—people, finances, processes, and customers—feels nearly impossible. Achieving results often requires emergency prioritization and mid-course corrections, challenging not only the business strategy but also the organization's capacity to adapt and execute effectively.

Challenges for Managers

It is evident that if we focus our attention on management levels, we will hear complaints that managers lack support from the organization's senior leadership, that all responsibilities rest on their shoulders, that employees are showing low levels of commitment, and that they need assistance to replace individuals and teams.

Human beings become increasingly complex when individuality is combined, and managers often feel that the more they depend on people, the more resistant those individuals become to work. Consequently, quality and time are impacted by the low performance of professionals.

Narratives emerge claiming that individuals from certain groups do not perform as well as those from other teams. This leads to various comparisons based on personal experiences and beliefs, creating space for unconscious biases and targeted accusations. In times of crisis, comparisons arise regarding the productivity of men versus women, individuals from different regions or social classes, and even between groups with varying educational backgrounds and skills. This dynamic can escalate to the point of pitting individual talents and competencies against one another.

In an attempt to correct imperfections, managers call for stricter policies to enforce discipline, becoming more coercive and directive. Depending on the circumstances, they may try to shape the ways tasks are performed based on the successes of their own past experiences. They increasingly seek to demonstrate task execution formats to ensure employees reach the same potential they themselves once achieved.

This heightened emphasis on discipline and rigid methodologies creates a certain distance between managers and employees, opening the door for other social actors directly connected to the workplace, such as union leaders, to emerge and spark conflicts. Unintentionally, employees turn to formal entities for fairness and balance, seeking to reclaim their rights due to poor communication and a lack of trust in management. This often results in an increase in legal disputes and intervention by protective authorities. Managers then begin to view employees as diverging from work obligations and influencing others negatively, reinforcing the belief that low efficiency and human factors are the root of all organizational problems.

To make matters worse, conflicts with coworkers, colleagues from other departments providing services, or even customers, who often seem to exist solely to create obstacles, further complicate matters. These conflicts create barriers and delays in process execution. What becomes most apparent in organizations is the finger-pointing, with blame being assigned to others for mistakes. This behavior fosters relationships with low trust levels and results in significant losses due to a lack of synergy and collaboration.

The Challenge is People

The crisis scenario directly influences people's perceptions and beliefs about organizations. They recognize the problems affecting each company and assign responsibility to senior leadership and managers.

Complaints about low autonomy and lack of recognition become the recurring theme in conversations among professionals. They lament the unavailability of resources and criticize senior leadership for inefficiency in defining vision and strategic positioning, arguing that processes, communication, and corporate guidelines are confusing.

They also point to a lack of evaluation when choosing leaders and managers, claiming that hiring and promotion policies are based on favoritism, following a "stacked deck" principle, and that talent is not given opportunities to perform or grow professionally within the organization.

The relationship between people and the company is seen as purely financial, aimed solely at achieving business goals, with individuals viewed as mere numbers in the broader ecosystem.

The greater the perception that the corporate system does not value people, the lower the degree of contribution to collective success. People hold their managers accountable for how they run the business and lead teams, leading to social criticism of the role of "boss" in all environments—within their discussion circles, employees attribute the worst adjectives to their managers.

I am often asked what to do when managers exhibit toxic leadership styles that destroy people's intent to do their best, reducing teams to mere task-doers, devoid of purpose and motivation, and ultimately draining the workplace of morale.

A Problem for Everyone

You have likely identified with many of the situations described so far and may even experience them in your own company. All these issues stem from what Lederman Consulting & Education[2] classified as the seven most common business problems: lack of member engagement and dissatisfaction; unsatisfactory work deliverables; a negative work environment; lack of goals or planning to achieve them; lack of transparency in decisions; inflexibility; and, finally, poor knowledge management.

If we analyze these problems from a generalized perspective, we can identify a common root: they are all related to people.

This is why billions of dollars are invested annually to shift people management from the quadrant of business vulnerabilities to the quadrant of expansion and prosperity. In 2019 alone, over $300 billion was invested in the corporate training market, and exponential growth in this investment is expected over the next decade.[3]

The scenarios we live in and the challenges we face always come with particularities that are difficult to manage. Therefore, I find it beneficial to present the arguments I hear from each of our business sectors to better understand the challenges that cause anxiety for most of us.

However, it seems our efforts are insufficient to succeed with this unique variable, which is heavily influenced by identities and capable of extraordinary results.

The key to understanding these challenges is realizing that all individuals, at every organizational level, dream and aspire to find solutions so that everyone can succeed and live their best personal and professional experiences through work. But the significant challenge still echoes everywhere with the question: "How can we change all of this?"

We know there is a solution, and we can give better meaning to the perfect alignment between senior leadership, managers, and employees, enabling organizations to operate more efficiently and meet societal expectations. To achieve this, we must reformulate our models and ensure that business environments also fulfill their evolutionary role in better integrating society.

Every enterprise deserves a brilliant journey focused on prosperity and longevity. Being an investor or entrepreneur always presents a significant challenge of social transformation, which is not only about our ability to make businesses succeed in terms of management practices but also about understanding our social commitment and what we are genuinely delivering to individuals.

Our solution, in addition to meeting the needs of people in this world, also impacts the entire ecosystem through our operational model and influence across various societal areas.

The greater our growth, the more we influence people's lives, delivering—through our well-structured processes, products, and services, rooted in the pillars of people, clients, processes, and finances—value that benefits society and exceeds expectations. All of this shapes lifestyles, standards, and humanity's ability to improve each day.

The significant challenge for all of us is understanding how we can do this brilliantly, adhering to the natural laws of humanity and transforming the future through today's business actions.

Yes, there are ways to succeed. We have real examples that demonstrate the superior performance of some organizations compared to others that insist on maintaining traditional management models. Therefore, the time has come to uncover these mysteries and make prosperity available to everyone.

How can we resolve the existential and belonging crises professionals face within organizations? How can corporate culture provide solutions at all levels and lead to the improvement of people, processes, and growth across all dimensions? What is missing in our strategy, and how can we execute it with high engagement levels from everyone involved?

The need to overcome management challenges arises at all levels and affects all groups, directly impacting the social system. This occurs both through the influence organizations exert on the environment in which they operate and the influences they receive from the same environment in which they are embedded.

**The greater we become,
the more we influence people's lives
by delivering, through our well-structured
practices
in processes, products, and
services—rooted in the pillars of
people management, clients, processes, and
finances—something that benefits society and
ensures that outcomes
exceed expectations.**

CHAPTER 2

CHALLENGES FOR TRANSFORMATION

Breaking Taboos and Creating Meaning in Work

Every day, as a people manager, I search for transformative solutions to help individuals find their paths and address complaints about the difficulties of navigating crises and problems that hinder organizational performance. In these environments, I often meet people expressing dissatisfaction, making it clear why engagement and job satisfaction indicators remain so low.

When I ask these professionals questions to understand what is truly happening in their work and the business, I often encounter a host of adversities that seem almost insurmountable. However, these conversations frequently reveal cold, empty concepts about performance and process, highlighting that we've automated our discourse and lost sight of the purpose behind our existence and actions, falling into what I call the abyss of social conformity.

The greatest crisis we face is not political or economic—though I do not wish to downplay the magnitude and impact of those scenarios—but a **crisis of meaning**. We have lost ourselves in a historical context of achievements and power, failing to recognize what we are doing with humanity's greatest potential: consciousness.

We seek linear, logical solutions to workplace problems, forgetting that humanity has reached its current stage through adaptability and a boundless perspective on the world. We've learned from nature's lessons, breaking away from conventional patterns we imposed on ourselves.

I often imagine how our first steps as humans unfolded in the past, overcoming challenges posed by highly efficient predators capable of wiping out our species. I think about a baby, so fragile, developing defenses against predators only in adolescence. In ancient times, with little developed intelligence, the risk of death and extinction loomed constantly.

I propose a hypothesis: in our earliest days, we decided to stick together to increase our chances of survival. We quickly discovered we are social and collaborative beings.

But staying together wasn't enough—our bodies needed energy to survive. Some members of the group ventured out to gather fruits or hunt for food. During this period, survival was a literal quest, as not everyone who left the group returned.

It was as though life resided within the community we left behind, and we ventured out in search of the resources necessary to sustain it. This was about life—or, more accurately, beyond life—facing challenges greater than our desires, with death often an unexpected outcome.

Over time, work began to take on the connotation of survival **(sur + vival)**. Gradually, we separated the notion of survival from what we called life itself. Much later, this division would evolve into the concept of work-life balance, seeking equilibrium between the good and the bad, which forms the true structure of our existence.

In the earliest days of survival—what we now term work—expressions like **"to take the bull by the horns," "no pain, no gain,"** and **"every dog has his day"** were quite literal and made sense in the formation of human society. Thousands of years later, these beliefs and customs still influence us. So, I ask: Where are today's bulls? What keeps us repeating these phrases? Could it be bosses? Employers? Clients?

We've adopted such a harsh view of work and survival that we've stopped noticing how **the act of "setting out" has shaped who we are today**. It's true: from the beginning, we've needed to develop skills, tools, and processes to enhance our existence. Yet these very processes have distanced us from the "why." Processes have been defined and applied, placing us in an unprecedented cycle of repetition that I call social conformity—a cycle that makes us forget why we do what we do.

The key fact is that, according to a Gallup study4, fewer than 15% of people worldwide are engaged in their work. These individuals experience emotional suffering at work, while the remaining 85%—including managers and business owners—underperform, feel deeply dissatisfied with results, worry about external scenarios, and rely on antiquated management models in a constant struggle against crises and losses.

Global Engagement

According to another Gallup survey5 conducted across 142 countries, approximately 1/8 of workers (equivalent to around 180 million people) are engaged in their jobs and more likely to make positive contributions to their organizations.

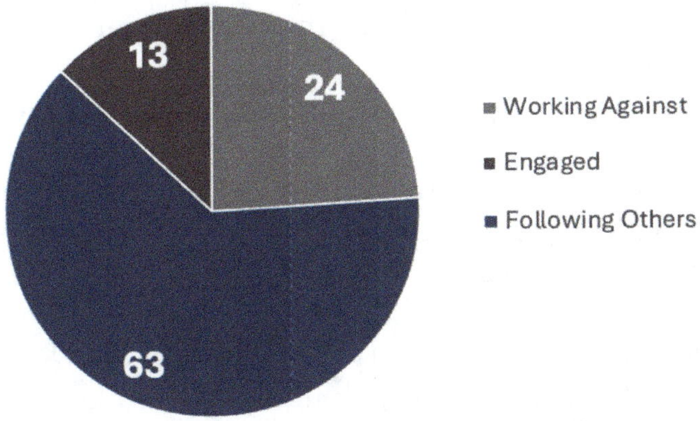

The same survey revealed that engagement levels also vary by region. The United States and Canada lead the ranking with 29% engaged workers, followed by Australia and New Zealand with 24%.

The topics of “boss” and “work” rank among the top five themes in social conversations. When people gather in groups at places like bars, restaurants, or sports venues, the majority discuss how their work environment negatively impacts their lives. These conversations often include comments about a mythical figure called "the boss," who seems to steal people’s happiness and turn their days into a living hell.

Globally, over 50% of the 500 largest companies listed in the 2000 Fortune ranking have disappeared 6. Among them were businesses from all sectors, including technology companies, which, despite modernization and creative environments, also lacked the resilience to survive.

If these prominent organizations from the Fortune list have vanished, imagine the fate of countless other companies worldwide that make up the vast majority of employers.

In the last twenty years, we have undergone a silent but significant transformation in the business environment and the ways work is performed.

Most organizations worldwide are composed of micro, small, and medium-sized companies with fewer than 1,000 employees. In Brazil, for instance, small businesses employ 70% of the workforce 7, a remarkably high number that cannot be ignored. For this reason, I strongly believe these companies will assume a new role in society.

Some people argue that nothing will change and that business practices will remain the same: individuals selling their time to contribute to something they do not believe in, chasing power, and pursuing financial achievements to one day enjoy the fruits of their efforts—if, by then, they still have the time and energy to do so.

Considering that in twenty years, 50% of the world's largest companies have ceased to exist, along with a similar proportion of smaller businesses, I say to those who believe nothing will change: today's market has been reinvented by 50% new companies. With the rapid acceleration of change driven by technology, new players will emerge at an even faster pace.

There are two primary ways a business can cease to exist. The first stems from the arrogance of its leaders, who fail to recognize that the world's needs are changing and that they must offer new solutions. Instead, they blame the market, competitors, government, and external factors, refusing to see that their offerings are no longer relevant while new solutions are being introduced.

None of this prevented the decline of these economic giants. The people who worked in these environments have moved on to other organizations, and other suppliers now deliver products and services to the clients of those vanished companies. For the most part, these organizations belong to history, and few will remember them in the near future—except perhaps for those extensively

I don't intend to delve deeply into the discussion of human evolution and the phases of achievements that have led us to where we are today—repeating meaningless patterns and living unhappily while hoping to someday connect with our happiness and what we might call a true life. It's remarkable how human beings, capable of spending their entire existence trying to discover if there is life after death, often forget to ask whether we have life before death.

studied by consultants and researchers or nostalgically recalled by former employees clinging to memories of "the good old days," sometimes resisting both the present and future projects.

Among these defunct companies, there is another group: those that "imploded" due to internal issues. This includes cases like Enron, once one of the largest oil conglomerates in the world, whose founder Kenneth Lay and CEO Jeffrey Skilling were convicted of conspiracy and fraud. 8 Despite all efforts, they lost sight of their core business in the pursuit of productivity and profitability. They created toxic environments, fueled scarcity-driven mindsets, and rigidly adhered to blind management practices.

These companies failed to nurture their ecosystems, forming relationships with employees, suppliers, and clients based solely on financial interests, with exploitation at the core. Customers became targets, employees were treated as resources, and suppliers were viewed as opportunities for cost reduction.

The companies clinging to 20th-century models focused on exploitative profitability are disappearing, along with the public that once valued wealth accumulation as a source of power. Societal values are shifting. According to the Gallup 9 study "The Brazilian Workforce Through the Lens of Engagement," the main current causes of employee disengagement are poor relationships with leadership, lack of employee recognition, outdated infrastructure, and misalignment between personal and professional values.

Humanity's greatest phenomenon is its ability to reinvent itself with each new generation. These new generations benefit from the evolutionary process of those before them and recognize the need to establish new ways of living and relating to one another. They break past paradigms and bring an evolved mechanism of human adaptation to the ongoing evolutionary process.

In the past fifty years, new generations of businesses have begun to emerge, and society has redefined its expectations for relationships with organizations, forcing the creation of new contractual dynamics. Communities of people seeking a new way to work are forming daily. Work has become an integral part of life for individuals who seek purpose and environments where happiness indices are a reality.

At an unprecedented pace, new businesses are being introduced to the world, already aligned with society's evolving desires and standards. Meanwhile, the old framed mission, vision, and values statements hanging on office walls remain in place, along with discussions on quality and safety standards.

However, a new word is gaining strength in these conversations: purpose. Alongside it comes the growing emphasis on valuing the ecosystem in which the organization operates and questioning the role of leadership.

**Considering everything we've discussed so far and the emergence of new management models, the key question is: What is the new business model,
and how can companies take on a new, meaningful role in people's lives?**

How can a company's purpose drive engagement and integrate work as a meaningful part of employees' lives, fostering healthy experiences and contributing to building a better society?

Does the world of work have a solution? What are we doing to ensure that excellence truly holds meaning in our lives?

CHAPTER 3

WHEN EVERYTHING IS CHAOTIC, WHERE DO YOU BEGIN?

The First Steps to Driving Significant Change

Starting the transformation by understanding the organization's purpose and mission would be ideal for initiating meaningful change. However, as we've seen, many environments face significant challenges in fostering engagement, earning trust, and adopting leadership styles that inspire people to achieve their dreams and evolve daily.

I share the same eagerness to discuss how to build a purpose that connects everyone to a cause greater than individual goals. But first, I need to address the emergency actions for those facing major crises and operating in environments plagued by a lack of engagement.

We must remember that engagement is scarce in the business world. Many people do not believe companies can provide healthy environments for them. Therefore, understanding what needs to be done and the power of small actions to change this reality is reassuring for those who still have a long way to go.

No step can be taken without first believing in the importance of having a clear purpose—one that shows people **why the organization exists in the world and how it serves society**. As Viktor Frankl stated in his book Man's Search for Meaning 10, quoting Heikel, "Those who have a 'why' to live can bear almost any 'how.'" This is why we cannot underestimate the power of purpose.

Another factor we will explore in future chapters is the importance of leadership style. Leadership is a fundamental element that **can positively impact up to 70% of employee satisfaction within an organization**. 11

You might be wondering: if purpose is so essential and leadership has such a significant influence on transformation, why focus first on small actions that have less impact on overall satisfaction?

The truth is, we must address purpose, leadership development, and the strengthening of our engagement pillars simultaneously. However, to ignite a movement, **we must first understand the pillars of each culture, the aspirations of its people, and how we can set an example that proves the transformations will be genuine and that everyone involved truly matters to the organization**.

Face the chaos with a simple and surprising first step

The Power of Active Listening

Listening to people and understanding their needs is the first step toward transformation. While we'll discuss specific actions, we must also address leadership behaviors as a way to break down organizational structures and patterns. By connecting with people on a deeper level, we can uncover their challenges: What obstacles prevent them from doing their work effectively? How can we gather their best ideas for performing tasks in ways that feel most appropriate to them?

Acting with simplicity may seem easy, but it often triggers self-sabotaging thoughts like "I already know this." However, it takes courage to execute what is simple and to admit that **it's not what we know that transforms the world, but what we do**. Execution is the key to all the changes we wish to see in the world around us. Ironically, **implementing simplicity can be incredibly challenging**. We often gravitate toward complex procedures to assert control, define mechanisms, and do things our way, largely because society fears listening to others and dealing with the awareness such openness generates.

Breaking barriers and establishing channels of dialogue helps us discover people's aspirations. But merely listening isn't enough; we must understand why people struggle to perform their best, acknowledge inefficiencies, and identify clear actions to address them. This mapping is the first step toward creating a culture of trust. When we address basic issues, like replacing heavy, outdated equipment with more user-friendly tools, people notice that our actions are genuine and that we truly care about their needs.

Many procedures exist as they are simply because someone authoritatively decided so. However, the people working within these processes often know how they could be improved and can offer meaningful suggestions.

This may sound obvious, but in most workplaces, arrogance, cost-containment policies, or a lack of dialogue with frontline workers lead to employees being subjected to tasks they don't believe in. They are often forced to do the work against their will, and then criticized for being uncommitted.

The first step toward transforming the work environment is to believe that everyone comes to work each day intending to give their best. Yet, when they encounter barriers, a lack of active listening, or, worse, disrespect, they feel undervalued. This triggers the law of reciprocity: people give back what they perceive they are receiving. And the energy returned is often the worst kind, as people reflect the lack of value they feel from the organization.

A common fear among managers regarding open dialogue is that employees will unleash a torrent of complaints, creating a "wall of lamentation." It's important to understand that complaints are a form of repeated clamor. We must approach these conversations in a way that moves from expressing grievances to collaboratively seeking solutions and realizing aspirations.

We need to improve our questioning skills. In my mentoring sessions with managers, I often hear them ask questions like, "What are you dissatisfied with?" or "What's wrong here, and what can we improve?" These questions tend to encourage complaints and take the focus away from actionable solutions. Instead, we should ask about **the challenges people face, their discomforts, and how they believe their tasks could be improved. What's missing in the work environment that prevents them from performing at their best every day?**

Such questions open up a greater potential for responses that enhance team performance and, consequently, their satisfaction with their work.

My observations may sound simple or trivial, but I regularly encounter research that confirms knowing what to do is not enough to achieve excellent people management and leadership in organizations. Most people fail to act, procrastinate, or lack the organization needed to make things happen. 12 I hear inspiring speeches during interviews, meetings, and conversations with business leaders. However, when I visit the frontline of these companies, I often discover that these beautiful speeches never reach the employees. If they did, they would undoubtedly create change.

Effectively conveying a message to all involved generates commitment.

At times, when progress fails to yield positive results, people begin to complain, and we must provide quick responses. If listening is not active, we risk being betrayed by our own rhetoric, failing to realize that, beyond complaints, grievances often carry suggestions derived from previous work environments. This could lead to the danger of becoming a poorly executed copy of another organization.

Benchmarking—researching activities in other companies—is a common practice in the market but can sometimes mislead us. It reinforces the principle of social conformity when we adopt what **everyone else is doing without understanding why we are doing it**. We should recognize and learn from the remarkable practices of others to enrich our knowledge and enhance organizational creativity. However, these practices must be adapted to align with our unique culture and the specific needs of our company's current situation.

Surprise people with actions inspired by dialogue. Such actions not only drive improvements in the organization but also make people feel valued and motivated.

I want to share a practice I implemented that produced impressive results in several projects. It helped build trust in our initiatives and served as a model for shaping best practices tailored to the culture of the companies where we were working.

Be remarkable

I call this activity remarkable because it has the power to introduce approaches that people may never have imagined. The exercise involves four stages: basic, expected, desired, and remarkable. It can be applied to any project, but for clarity, let's use the example of planning the launch of a new gas station. Imagine we are embarking on this venture together—a business model familiar and utilized by many.

What is basic for a gas station? Likely, you'd suggest basic elements like the product: gasoline, and diesel fuel, along with a fuel pump, canopy, underground tanks, and a suitable plot of land.

What is expected from a gas station? High-quality products and services, fair pricing, credit and debit card payment options, and a convenience store are likely considerations that come to mind.

What is desired from a gas station? Competitive pricing, exceptional customer service, amenities like tire pressure calibration, a car wash, a tire repair shop, glass cleaning, and a loyalty program.

Now, imagine a **remarkable** gas station. It needs to be truly outstanding—unlike any you've encountered before. Can you envision it? Let's build this concept together. However, what's remarkable today may not remain so for long, as society evolves and competitors adapt, reshaping their concepts to meet new expectations. To maintain the status of remarkable, reinvention is essential to avoid blending into the mainstream, where what was once innovative becomes standard.

Picture this: You pull into a gas station on a crisp, sunny day, ready to refuel your car. The station is immaculately clean, and the pumps are well-maintained and easy to navigate. You step out of your car and swipe your credit card at the pump, effortlessly selecting your preferred grade of gasoline. As the pump hums softly, filling your tank, you glance over and notice a small but inviting convenience store.

Curious, you walk inside. The space is modern and welcoming, with a well-stocked selection of coffee, chilled drinks, snacks, and even a few fresh baked goods that fill the air with a comforting aroma. There's a seating area with plush chairs and USB charging stations—perfect for a quick recharge, both for you and your devices.

Once your tank is full, you return to your car and notice a complimentary windshield cleaning station with fresh squeegees and cleaning solution. Before heading back on the road, you take a moment to clean your windshield and check your tire pressure using the free air pump conveniently located nearby.

The entire experience feels effortless and thoughtful, as if the

We must remember that engagement is scarce in the business world. Many people do not believe that companies can provide healthy environments for them. Therefore, understanding what needs to be done and recognizing the power of small actions to change this reality is reassuring for those who still have a long journey ahead.

station was designed with you in mind. Though there's no attendant greeting you or handling the service, the station's setup and amenities make it clear that your time and comfort are valued. You leave feeling refreshed, your car ready for the road, and silently think to yourself, "Why can't every gas station be like this?"

Does that surprise you? If you've never encountered a place like this, it probably does. This premium service might come with a higher price tag, but many customers would still prefer this experience. When customers perceive your product or service as an exceptional experience, competitors pale in comparison.

Now, think about the complaints and resource requests you've heard from your team. How can you surprise them? What can you do right now to make the experience extraordinary for everyone? Ask yourself and your team: What is basic in this activity, resource, or project? What is expected by our customers? What is desired? And how can we, with the resources available, make the experience remarkable?

This exercise is simple yet powerful. It prevents us from merely copying solutions that worked for others, ensuring our strategies align with our culture and current needs.

Listening attentively and acting swiftly will significantly impact perceptions, building a following for transformation efforts. By demonstrating genuine care and proactive solutions, we strengthen trust and inspire change.

Organizational challenges often stem from overly complex solutions that fail to meet people's needs, implemented simply because "that's how it's done elsewhere." As leaders, we must simplify our approaches to recognition, communication, celebration, development, and collaboration. It's challenging but essential to break free from the conformity that stifles innovation.

In the early stages of transformation, gaining the trust of your first followers is crucial. Nurture them, providing support and assurance that your actions are genuine and that others can trust the future you're building. Your first follower sets the tone for the influence of your leadership, followed by the next, and the next. This process relies on consistency and alignment between your actions and words. Inspire through action, and you'll pave the way for enduring trust and transformation.

Surprise people with actions driven by meaningful dialogue, as these actions not only drive improvements within the company but also leave individuals feeling motivated and valued.

What have you been doing that surprises the people around you?

Is there something you can do to inspire trust in your mission among your team?

Is there a simple action you can take right now that will spark thoughts about the better future you aim to create?

CHAPTER 4

WHY DOES YOUR BUSINESS EXIST AND WHAT DOES IT DO FOR THE WORLD?

The reason we do what we do every day is the inner strength, recognized as the cause we stand for.

Some people claim that purpose is just a buzzword in organizational settings. I am often challenged to explain how purpose can be defined and what benefits it offers to professionals working in an organization with a clear mission to serve society.

Through research on the evolution of businesses and an effort to understand why 50% of Fortune companies no longer exist, it became evident that there are five levels of companies in the world.

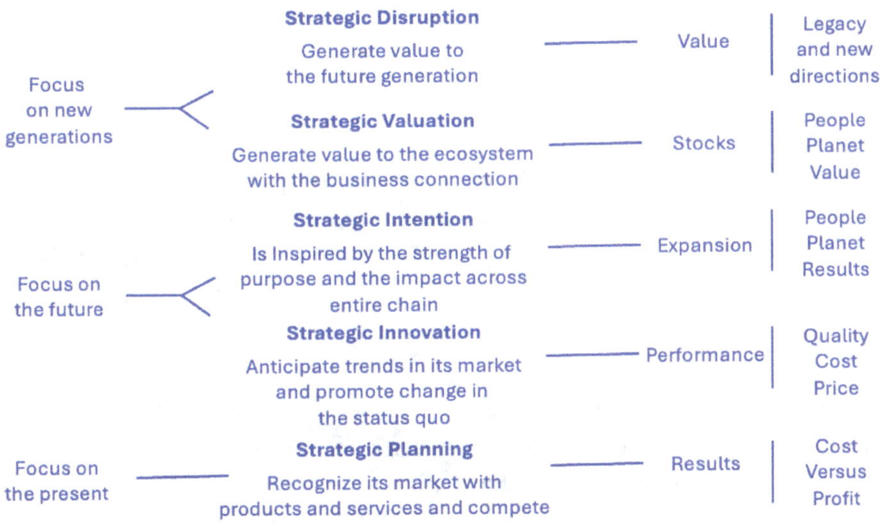

Strategic Disruption
Generate value to the future generation
Value
Legacy and new directions
Focus on new generations
Strategic Valuation
Generate value to the ecosystem with the business connection
Stocks
People Planet Value
Strategic Intention
Is Inspired by the strength of purpose and the impact across entire chain
Expansion
People Planet Results
Focus on the future
Strategic Innovation
Anticipate trends in its market and promote change in the status quo
Performance
Quality Cost Price
Focus on the present
Strategic Planning
Recognize its market with products and services and compete
Results
Cost Versus Profit

Strategic Planning: Recognizes its market through products and services and competes. The foundation of the business is supported by a focus on results, with the core equation of the enterprise rooted in the cost-revenue relationship. The most frequent discourse in this organizational model is: "We need to reduce costs to sustain our results." The primary focus of this business model is on the present.

Strategic Innovation: Anticipates market trends and drives change in the status quo. Its foundation is supported by a transition from focusing solely on results to emphasizing performance, introducing the relationship between quality, cost, and benefit. A language centered on customer focus begins to emerge, although the policy still positions the customer as a target rather than a solution. The prevailing discourse in this organizational model is competitive, asserting that "it's necessary to get ahead of the competition." Once this advantage diminishes, the business enters a decline in growth as others replicate its model. At this point, the company returns to the competitive cycle in the strategic planning stage.

Strategic Intention: Draws inspiration from the power of purpose and its impact throughout the entire chain. Its foundation is built on the company's reason for existing and its way of serving the world and society. It prioritizes creating meaning so that everyone in its chain can contribute, recognizes individual purpose, and seeks to integrate organizational values with personal values. The focus is directed toward the future, emphasizing contributions that positively impact people, the planet, and outcomes, fostering a desire to propose value to the world. The term "for what purpose" gains prominence in this organizational model, and people begin to be seen as the center of the business, promoting the idea that "the business of business is people." The results take into account engagement levels and happiness indexes at work.

Strategic Valuation: Creates value for the ecosystem through the enterprise's connection. The entire business is designed to serve the world in a clear and specific way, seeking recognition as a conscious platform that clearly resolves a societal need. Its actions have an immediate impact that influences future generations, with a value proposition that is evident to society at large.

The enterprise's activities address a global need while maintaining clear economic objectives. It generates financial resources throughout its chain, with social impact integrated into its model. This often includes practices that promote equality, combat poverty and hunger, or address other specific needs, aligned with the UN's sustainable development goals. The communication strategy typically begins with the question: "**What global need can my business address while remaining prosperous?**"

Strategic Disruption: Creates value for future generations. It breaks paradigms upheld for decades, establishing new ways for humanity to overcome challenges. It anticipates trends and, after its emergence, sets new standards for behavior or needs, disrupting habits and customs. The level of innovation extends beyond products and services, embedding itself into social models, dismantling societal biases, and establishing new norms. The business model generates absolute value for the world, inspired by building a legacy and charting new courses for humanity. It reflects on the question: "**What kind of world do we want to leave for future generations, and how can we help achieve this transformation?**"

Understanding the levels of businesses was essential to recognizing that the organizations disappearing from our society today are the same ones that succeeded for a long time in the past by focusing on the present and managing the cost-revenue equation diligently. Similarly, while innovation-driven environments have succeeded in their strategies, many others failed to survive market challenges. Workers, though satisfied with financial performance and compensation practices, often felt economically exploited, fostering relationships driven purely by financial interests. This left their loyalty vulnerable to any offer that exceeded this transactional model.

Respect for human beings was limited to the transactional basis of relationships, sidelining emotional connections, as companies only valued rational contributions. Workers sought reciprocity to balance this rationality.

We live in a world where people perceive everything around them as definitive; they proudly proclaim their intelligence and propagate discourse as if they fully understand humanity and society. Yet the most remarkable aspect of our social ecosystem is that everything we create is destined for obsolescence within its historical context. What we value and deem fundamental today will cease to exist. New generations will transform everything into a better context, questioning everything we've done for the world and how we've conducted ourselves.

Take, for instance, products like typewriters, floppy disks, DVDs, and other societal solutions—each had its life cycle. Without adaptation and evolution, manufacturers of such items were forgotten. The same principle applies to business models and management practices.

Commitments for Reimagining Business Models:

- **Embrace a sense of belonging to a greater cause.**
- **Exercise creative and innovative potential to take ownership of progress.**
- **Listen and share the best of one's essence.**
- **Be challenged with questions that expand awareness.**
- **Work as an expression of talent and vocation to pursue a mission.**
- **Understand that everything is interconnected, and systemic effects are inevitable.**

This historical overview of business scenarios and operational models reveals that strategies alone are insufficient to ensure organizations' survival in the future. Reinvention and principles—like the Buddhist philosophy of evolving and serving—are reshaping how we lead companies. New questions challenge paradigms and inspire change. We must adjust our practices to embrace and accelerate adaptation, serving the new generations poised to lead enterprises. This equilibrium will integrate work as part of life, no longer a mere path to survival.

Creating a Journey to Transform the Universe While Respecting Our Pace

Respecting the evolutionary steps of people and culture is essential to maintain credibility and progress in a transformation strategy. Knowing where we want to go is indispensable, but **the greatest villain of all strategies is the anxiety to reach our desired destination and the difficulty in dealing with frustrations that make us skip steps.**

If your company were to disappear today, what void would it leave in the world that no other company could fill?

Does the product or service you deliver address a need that goes beyond its own function?

Are you able to fill the emptiness of meaning within people by explaining the significance your business holds for the world?

The **From Listening to Growth method** (listen, understand, execute, standardize, energize, and evolve) will make a significant difference in guiding the transformation strategy and help you recognize progress at each stage of the plan.

When we focus solely on the long-term objective and the desired destination, we risk losing momentum due to the perceived long distance. Major challenges can erode our confidence in achieving them, making it harder to keep people energized for a long journey.

We can direct our attention as follows: establish our purpose, define the overarching goal, and work on smaller milestones, applying the From Listening to Growth method step by step in each phase.

Listening

As previously mentioned, creating opportunities for meaningful dialogue reinforces the first axis of executing short-term actions because listening is a key factor in gathering the most valuable contributions from people.

A critical warning for those embarking on this journey is to avoid doing things out of obligation or without genuine intent. It's important to steer clear of standardizing or formalizing something that should flow naturally. The goal is to create positive habits and enhance the capacity for dialogue. The From Listening to Growth method is also useful for changing small habits, meaning each step should be executed with a focus on improving current practices and refining them after evaluating the success of each cycle.

Some individuals, influenced by benchmarking, attempt to implement changes by scheduling fixed times and dates for dialogues. This approach risks reinforcing social conformity, potentially turning these interactions into forced routines. Over time, such practices may lead to mockery, as everyone recognizes it as "the scheduled chat with the managers." Beyond causing discomfort, this approach removes any sense of spontaneity. Be cautious when initiating conversations, as forcing these moments without a natural flow may make you the subject of jokes in hallways and break rooms.

According to a study by the American leadership company Zenger Folkman, 13 the key traits of exceptional listeners are: focusing on the other person, participating in the dialogue by offering suggestions, being open to criticism, creating a safe environment, and demonstrating empathy. As you can see, active listening is challenging, but developing new habits and committing to others will help you seize the opportunity to learn from professionals and their perspectives on various topics. Moreover, **every interaction is an opportunity to gain insights from diverse viewpoints, experiences, and contributions, which can lead to reevaluating beliefs and establishing new behavioral and thought patterns**.

Individual Dialogues: Foster one-on-one interactions in unplanned moments, treating these encounters as opportunities to learn and grow personally. These exchanges will be enriching and help strengthen your connections.

Collective Dialogues: Create moments for group dialogue outside of formal settings (like meetings). Encourage interactions free from rigid formats and use these experiences to learn from collective knowledge. Recognize the current context of the group and seek ways to enhance resources and processes, enabling members to perform their tasks more freely and effectively.

Understanding

It seems simple, but it's not. Our cognitive patterns often lead us to quickly recognize another person's speech, compare it to the patterns we already hold based on our life history and experiences, and immediately infer a response as if we already know everything the other person intends to convey. This is the mechanism of inference.

Indeed, we often translate everything the other person says into terms we already understand, assuming we have all the answers. Our greatest challenge, when striving to make the best impact on people's lives, is learning to let go of our paradigms and fully immerse ourselves in the other person's needs.

To facilitate this, it's essential to prioritize questions over answers. **The quality of the questions we ask will broaden our understanding, illuminate the other person's awareness of their own thoughts, feelings, and actions, and offer new perspectives of understanding.**

You may very well have the answer, but resist the urge to interrupt or impose it. Allow the other person to evolve with everything they are expressing. Let them participate in crafting the solution and take ownership of what they believe in.

Understanding is the art of internalizing the perspectives projected by the other person based on their life experience. By committing to them, we also give them the freedom to commit to the solution and to live their best selves in this shared journey.

Executing

We have identified what can be improved; now, we need to organize everything to execute what is possible with the resources we have. This will yield the first fruits of change. Scholars worldwide emphasize the importance of defining what, why, who, where, when, how, and how much for a successful action to be implemented—a method widely known today as 5W2H.

If we are aiming to change the standard, execution is essential to achieve new outcomes in everything we do and experience.

The understanding phase has deepened our commitment through the level of insight and empathy gained, while also bringing others along on the journey. Following this, it is time to manage the execution because we now have all the reasons to act.

In a culture with a low level of trust in execution, it is critical to define monitoring steps and consistently involve the people engaged in the action by asking them to manage and monitor progress. This collaborative approach ensures that we can track and evaluate the results together.

Standardizing

For people to recognize the new standard, we must ensure conformity so that understanding is clear and free of doubts.

The word "standardization" plays a crucial role in the education process, helping consolidate new habits, providing clarity to the changes we make, and serving as an excellent benchmark to measure success in the upcoming steps.

Rely on people to define the new approach and establish a solid foundation, enabling others to begin their projects and take their steps based on the new standard. Sharing this standard with as many people as possible facilitates its adoption. However, there's another essential factor to consider: other individuals also become involved in the change, recognizing the transformations as progress is made each day and moment.

Gradually, we expand the energy of execution, attracting more committed followers to the transformation of the environment.

Energizing

Better than introducing new practices that align with people's expectations and needs is recognizing the energetic momentum generated by positive changes and amplifying the benefits for everyone impacted by them.

The change curve, developed by Elisabeth Kübler-Ross to help individuals cope with loss and trauma, is widely utilized in the corporate world due to its cyclical nature, which affects confidence and human energy levels. 15 It is essential to closely observe people's behavior as they navigate significant changes to break cycles of negativity as quickly as possible.

Communicating the benefits of new practices in a positive manner and empowering people to understand how these changes impact their lives and work strengthens the leader's role as a communicator. This approach showcases the leader's inspiring influence in transforming the organizational climate and fostering a culture of engagement.

Publicly recognizing and thanking each individual for their contributions is the most effective way to nurture the leader's

The From Listening to Growth method is also useful for changing small habits. In other words, execute each step by refining what you do today and improve after understanding that each cycle has been completed.

followers, from the longest serving to the most recent. **A leader's success is not defined solely by their actions; how their followers or team members spread positive energy to others will determine the pace at which broader consciousness is achieved. This, in turn, accelerates the overall transformation process.**

Evolving

The world is in constant evolution, and our agility in improving what is new will determine the pace at which we transform the culture of engagement. After celebrating and establishing a new standard, the experiences we provide will shift people's expectations from "basic" to "desired" in the cycle of enchantment, moving closer to "extraordinary." Thus, it becomes essential to revisit these practices, break away from what we've built, and pursue a new standard.

The process of evolution requires detachment from everything we have created and delivered to the world. It calls for a return to the foundation of the transformation model—listening attentively and recognizing the next steps to take. Evolution in listening and understanding must continue, as deepening our approach and maintaining an open mind are critical to avoiding the plateau of "I've gone as far as I can." There will always be opportunities for new achievements and for delighting people.

Every transformation begins with systemic actions, and even a small decision can significantly impact many professionals, particularly in environments with low engagement. When nothing has been done, even the smallest step holds great value.

As we evolve, we realize that every detail matters, and these small gestures demonstrate through action that even little things carry immense significance. **This affirms that simplicity, while powerful, is not easy**. In truth, the details leave lasting marks on people's lives and create significant impacts.

The accumulation of daily actions forms the foundation and pillars of transformation. **Listening, understanding, executing, standardizing, energizing, and evolving** enable the progress we need. Over time, many small actions, perfectly executed, will lead to the achievement of greater objectives.

Sharing each step in the journey "from Listening to Growth" builds trust and reduces anxiety. However, meticulous monitoring is essential, as skipping even one of these steps can undermine progress, jeopardize evolution, and call all actions into question, ultimately eroding trust.

How do people feel
after spending time
in your presence?

How do you evoke in others
the feeling of being genuinely heard?

How do you
help people understand
how much you care about them?

How do you
inspire people to be
better after an
encounter with you?

CHAPTER 5

THE "WHY" IN PRACTICE

Unveiling the Paths to Discover Purpose

Probably you would tell me that, aware of what everyone is currently discussing, you already understood the importance of working for a cause. However, while in theory it's a simple concept to grasp, many companies struggle to define in practice what their purpose is. For this reason, I'll help you highlight your strength and outline some steps to identify an organization's purpose.

It is evident that in times of change within business environments, there are still numerous enterprises treating purpose as merely the essence of a phrase to support a marketing repositioning. This might work initially but let me remind you that while it's possible to deceive the market for a while, no one can deceive themselves for long. If the purpose doesn't resonate with you, believe me, the lack of authenticity will soon become apparent to others.

I observe that countless organizations attempt to define a purpose as a means to gain an advantage, reap the benefits provided by that purpose, and sustain their models while still focusing solely on profitability. They often use their message to mislead society and consumers.

It is crucial to note that, in this journey toward evolving business models, we are witnessing not only a new generation of organizations but also existing organizations repositioning their reason for being, making purpose their expression and their cause to exist. In doing so, they serve society more fully and intensely, championing a noble cause for all and transforming their service into a cycle of prosperity and transformation.

Purpose is not a goal. Many people confuse "living for a purpose or a cause" with "having a purpose or a cause to live off." Inspired by the book Vidas Vazias (Empty Lives) by Divaldo Franco, which discusses the importance of having a cause, 16 I understand that purpose is tied to the principle and transformation your business provides to the world.

Our organization will experience the full strength of its purpose when it achieves a balance between its reason for serving the world, the way it inspires people to live their best every day and desire to be part of the organization, and, finally, its promotion of a cycle of continuous evolution.

This allows individuals to feel the joy of achieving something admirable with daily excellence. It is as though people receive a call to join a cause and find inspiring leaders who foster their growth, ensuring they are constantly developing in all areas of life: intellectual, physical, social, psychological, and spiritual.

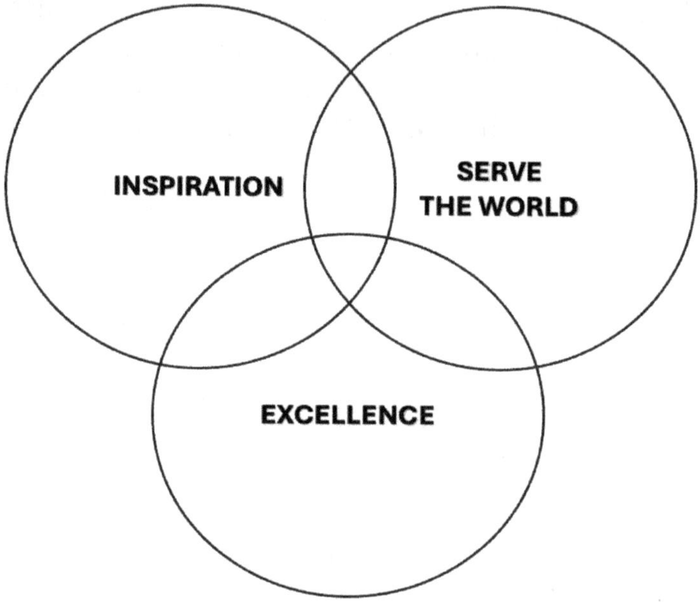

Few companies have a clear understanding of their mission and the benefits they bring to the world. To reflect on whether we have clear answers to this, we can utilize the **4 I's of organizational coherence with the world**.

The first "I" demands a commitment to **intention**. We need to answer, "Why do we exist?" and "What do we stand for?"

The second "I" highlights the necessity of a commitment to how we **inspire** those around us. We must have the competence to answer questions such as, "What value do we represent to the world?", "What do we offer people?", and "How do we influence their lives?"

Recognizing **identity** is essential to defining who we are and who we attract to represent us to the world. This leads us to the "I" that answers, "Who are we?" and, consequently, we must acknowledge, "Who will connect with us?", "What are our values?", and "What does our audience think, feel, and need?"

Finally, the "I" that defines our **image** to the world also deserves emphasis. It's crucial to have clear answers to questions like, "Who am I to everyone and to my market?", "What do those connected to me express?", and "What are the attributes that define us?"

If these questions are easily answered, the organization is likely highly evolved and clearly connected to the future needs of new generations. However, if the answers remain hidden behind uncertainty, one of the greatest attributes we must develop is the ability to ask powerful questions, encouraging reflection and moving organizations out of their comfort zone to drive prosperity and align with society's evolving needs.

We must shift the narrative that businesses exist solely to make money. While profit is undoubtedly important—fundamental for fueling cycles of prosperity and an indicator of business health and high profitability—I am not dismissing profit or critiquing capitalism. Instead, I believe every evolutionary process must consider all areas of contribution to ensure a business's sustainability, strengthening every link in the chain and fostering conscious growth.

According to performance metrics from Great Place to Work (GPTW)-certified companies, new business models focused on management awareness—ensuring the entire ecosystem benefits—yield profitability three times higher than those tracked by the S&P 500 (U.S. stock market). 17 Furthermore, companies recognized as great places to work exhibit average growth rates twice as high as those listed on the Worldwide Stock Exchange.

So how do we define the purpose of our organization? How do we understand the essence of our business and spread that intention? Many leaders panic when it comes to defining purpose, as if embarking on a quest for the unknown. However, the truth is that purpose already exists within the organization; the challenge lies in making it clear.

The first step is to **recognize the actions that define us**. Understanding what we currently do and how we bring our products and services to life is a good starting point for understanding who we are. We must also take the opportunity to identify whom we benefit and how we reach them to provide our best.

One of the best questions I ask teams is: "What are the world's pains that we help alleviate, and how do we do it so intuitively that even we struggle to notice?"

Having clarity about the world's problems and how we address them broadens our perspective on the benefits we create. For example, a synthetic reinforcement company for rubber may see itself as enhancing global safety through the quality of its products and services. However, deeper investigation might reveal that creating the best reinforcements for rubber isn't possible without a special focus on strengthening people. Therefore, the company must provide daily opportunities for human development, equipping individuals to better serve the world through their work, creating extraordinary products and services, and reinforcing society while building a better world.

Similarly, consider a bus driver. While many may view their role as merely operating a vehicle, a bus company's purpose is far greater. It connects people, facilitates dreams, and reduces distances—bringing humanity closer together.

We live to create solutions for society, and integrating people with those solutions fosters an alignment of aspirations and desires, inspiring a collective journey where everyone constantly strives for something greater.

Our intention spreads our vital energy and generates motivation for action. The greater the sense of purpose, the stronger the connection with what we do, and the greater the expansion of recognition and admiration for our daily work. **Everyone leaves their home each day with the dream of experiencing meaningful moments that foster growth, enabling them to perform at their best**.

The benefit we provide to society is a marvelous source of energy, and I believe this explains why so many people engage in volunteer work, dedicating their best talents without expecting anything in return, simply for the feeling of fulfilling their mission. Recognizing how and whom we are benefiting serves as a source of inspiration to continue on our journey.

Our sense of fulfillment materializes when we acknowledge that we are unique, accomplishing something extraordinary that brings good to others. Individuality in the execution of work within organizations is essential to feel our presence in what we build. We may perform similar tasks to others, but if we recognize that connecting with others provides them opportunities for growth, our sense of fulfillment and self-worth is amplified. This is why it is truly wonderful to acknowledge our individuality and the significance we hold as unique beings.

Kordsa, which ranked first in the Work Happiness Index (IFT) by Você S/A magazine in Brazil 18 in 2019, clearly understood at the time that its environment was more than just a place for work and production—it was where people came together daily to create unforgettable experiences for everyone present. Recognizing the message we represent to the world is fundamental in clarifying our purpose, our genuine intention, and our mission.

This is not about achieving a goal, making more money, or acquiring material possessions—it's about the sense of fulfillment through the habit of serving, bringing meaning and significance to life, and balancing and sustaining it with the power to generate prosperity.

In my view, the concept that best encapsulates the idea of finding purpose is Ikigai, which I learned from the inhabitants of Okinawa, Japan, and which has spread globally.

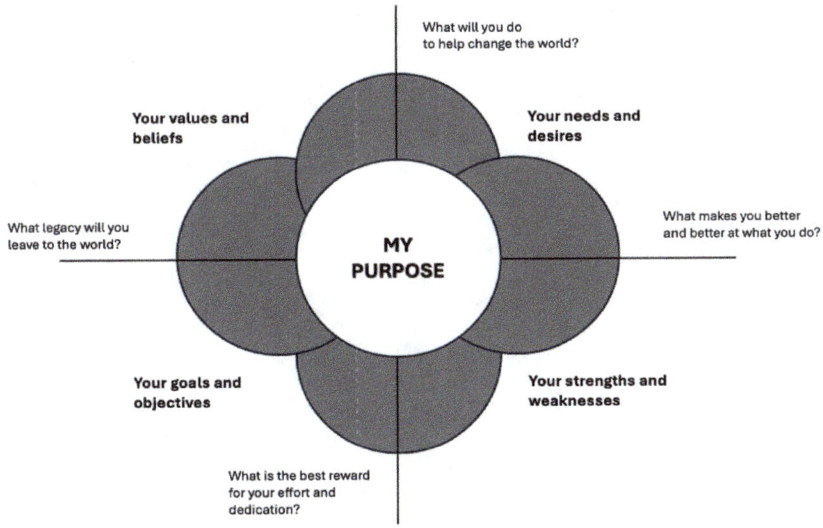

Understanding what we do every day to help change the world fosters profound organizational transformation. We must constantly repeat the phrase, "The business of businesses is people." Everything we create in this world should serve humanity and the planet.

Does your organization recognize the actions that contribute to making the world a better place?

How do we change people's lives?

Do we identify any alignment between what we do and the planet's needs?

Does our operational model support any of the UN's sustainable goals?

CHAPTER 6

WHAT IS CULTURE, AFTER ALL?

Defining Organizational Culture and Its Key Elements for Success

People often think of culture as something that emerges suddenly. They fail to consider that the term is originally derived from biology, where it represents how cells behave in a shared environment. While I could delve into the intricacies of this definition to remain true to its origins, our goal of understanding corporate engagement culture requires us to shift focus from biological nuances to analyzing organizational "cells."

The first element we must consider before exploring the synergy of factors that reinforce organizational culture is the environment. In an organization, it's the combination of people's behaviors that, when acting together with a degree of coherence and consistency, begins to form the organizational climate. Over time, this climate reinforces the organizational culture. Consequently, different environments can exhibit distinct characteristics, primarily because they are shaped by the people within them.

In the context of an organization, there are key drivers that, when clearly communicated and understood by all, significantly influence trends and shape organizational culture. These drivers are: **purpose, vision and people**.

Purpose

The primary factor for driving direction is **purpose**, as discussed in the previous chapter. It is essential to understand **why our organization exists and the difference it makes in the world.** Recognizing our purpose connects us to our cause. Identifying our reason for being is the starting point and defines what motivates us every day. However, we must also understand where we want to go.

Vision of the future

The organizational vision aims to define this destination, fulfilling the role of clarifying who we aspire to be once we have acquired all the attributes necessary to strengthen our cause in the world.

At this stage, we begin to recognize our expression and the qualities we wish to embody. We open our minds to identify the compass that will define the characteristics, virtues, and competencies we need to become the organization we envision for society.

The strategy starts to make sense: we now understand why we operate in this world and what our goals are to achieve our objectives. Next, it's time to outline the steps for this transformation.

People

If culture refers to how all the cells of an organism behave, and we are discussing the transformations we will implement in our organization, it is now time to identify the cells that make up the organization: the people, their talents, and what we will reinforce to strengthen our competencies and transform the current structure into the organization we aim to build.

The synergy among behaviors, driven by values, beliefs, and emotions, will foster the changes and alignment we seek, shaping, through our actions, what we represent, who we are, and the steps we take in favor of our cause.

This is the moment to recognize who is aligned with us, what their strengths are, how those strengths contribute to reinforcing the purpose, and how we will communicate to promote transparency in everything we do.

Each environment and organizational model encompasses a unique set of competencies and values that guide people in their day-to-day work. However, certain human factors—when absent—make it significantly harder to move forward. Here are five critical elements essential for fostering a strong sense of responsibility and commitment.

PASSION: The fuel of life

Like any other fuel, passion requires periodic refueling to ensure the highest level of energy. Think of it like your car—it needs gas, oil, electricity or any other power regularly, because if the tank runs empty, the car won't have the energy to move forward.

Yet, we often neglect to refuel our relationships, professional goals, interests in learning, and desires in life. If we don't nurture and cultivate our passion, we risk losing energy and giving up halfway through our journey.

Passionate people remain steadfast in their purpose. Recognizing your passions and actively cultivating them helps to build resilience and develop the skills needed to overcome challenges. When fueled by passion, obstacles become stepping stones, and the journey itself becomes as rewarding as the destination.

ADMIRATION: Seek out people who do admirable things and collaborate with them.

There are many people in the world who seek admiration and followers. However, the better approach is: "What did you do today that is admirable? How do you evaluate your work?"

Working alongside individuals who consistently strive to surprise with their work and enchant others makes a difference for the world and any business environment. Finding people who shape their own destinies and inspire both self-admiration and the admiration of others is crucial to achieving success.

The essential element to evoke admiration lies in your actions, accomplishments, and the transformations you create. Seeking admiration for the sake of recognition alone tends to build individuals who complain about not receiving the value they believe they deserve. On the other hand, those who are doers and achievers initiate the process of self-admiration, which naturally extends outward.

ATTITUDE: Having attitude is inherent to being human. Everyone has it.

The difference lies in the energy that attitude conveys. Some people face most of their moments with a positive attitude toward challenges, while others adopt a negative stance when confronted with problems. I don't expect to find individuals who always maintain a positive attitude, as I recognize our tendency toward balance. However, most people lean toward a particular type of attitude, and I prefer those inclined to bring a positive outlook and provide solutions.

A negative attitude keeps a person stuck in complaints—repeating grievances without taking action. On the other hand, those with a positive attitude may also acknowledge difficulties and challenges but quickly shift to seeking solutions.

A positive attitude represents movement.

TALENT: Seek talented individuals.

Talented individuals often seem called to live out a special mission. Some say talent is the ability to excel in something with extraordinary depth. While I deeply admire the depth that talent represents, we must broaden our perspective to recognize that talent is also about breadth.

In today's world, it's not enough to master a subject deeply without understanding the broader scope of our actions and their impact on others and the ecosystem. **Being the best means little if it doesn't benefit others, uplift our peers, or positively impact the world.** True talent lies not only in individual excellence but in the ability to create value for the collective.

COMPLEMENTARITY: United by Strengths and Diversity

Following the principle of breadth, it is essential to discuss complementarity: the evolution of teamwork.

In our professional journey, we've all collaborated on various projects with others, and this is not an isolated initiative. Throughout human history, countless examples demonstrate global synergy, involving individuals from diverse fields and locations.

We need to understand that strengths are distributed across people worldwide. For years, we've focused on overcoming weaknesses, as if the essence of evolution lay in eliminating our flaws. If your weakness is preventing you from expanding and evolving, it's worth addressing—because anything that freezes your champion potential must be resolved.

However, there is a transformative way to advance and become better for the world. It happens when we operate collectively and, even more significantly, when we recognize our strengths, connecting them with those of others to amplify success together.

Acknowledging strengths and putting them into collaborative action is the competitive advantage we will leave for future generations. By turning competitive potential into a collaborative movement, we're on the verge of reshaping the concept of work, reinforcing the belief that "together we are genuinely stronger."

Practicing Coherence, Consistency, and Trust

We can observe different cultural models across various organizations. However, what must not be tolerated is a lack of coherence, consistency, and trust that arises from misalignment in environments where marketing and politically correct narratives are prioritized, but the internal reality contradicts what is being promoted.

After deciding which people will connect with us, we need to establish practices and policies that reinforce our pursuit of purpose. This involves embarking on a journey to become what we aspire to be according to our vision, while valuing our essence and leveraging our strengths in the desired direction.

The significant challenge for organizations is to avoid mimicking models and slogans adopted from other companies based on what some senior executives aspire to become. Often, these leaders fail to demonstrate coherence, resulting in the establishment of lofty goals that are detached from reality. This happens because the defined practices are contrary to the expected behaviors.

For example, setting high levels of process security does not inherently foster creativity. Similarly, aggressive compensation policies aimed at showcasing competitiveness do not align with a collaborative culture. Yet, it is common for senior management to

**The synergy between behaviors,
driven by values, beliefs,
and emotions, will foster
the changes and alignment
we aim for and will define,
based on our actions,
what we represent, who we are,
and the measures we take
in support of our cause.**

define apparent values and attempt to reinforce them with contradictory policies, as if one could consume a food item and keep it intact.

Human resource management practices need to be revisited to reflect the strategic directions that will support behaviors aligning with the organization's vision and purpose.

Promoting Synergy

In the end, it is the behavior of leadership that will determine whether the entire ecosystem operates in synergy with what has been planned.

Synergy represents the common alignment of energy, and it is the leader's responsibility to ensure this alignment in practice by living the organization's values intensely and spreading them so that everyone can drive a revolution in the environment and pursue the purpose.

Yes, it is a fact that the leader can dictate the success or failure of a culture. However, we will address this subject in a dedicated chapter, where the true essence of leadership will take center stage.

How clear is the level of purpose in your organization?

Is the vision properly aligned and reinforcing the purpose and mission?

Do behaviors, supported by values, beliefs, feelings, and emotions, strengthen the alignment of actions to achieve the vision?

Is there coherence, consistency, and trust between the management tools and people's behaviors?

The Blindness of Leaders and the Ghost of Failure

Our inability to take risks and our fear of failure lead us toward a management model that lacks efficiency and immobilizes us. People progress in their careers every day, and success often becomes failure's closest companion because it fosters a fear of losing what has been achieved. We panic at the thought that a single action might jeopardize everything we've built.

The business world has adopted a standardized format with its own specific language. Anyone who strays from this mode of communication risks exclusion from this exclusive "business world." It's astonishing how quickly we adopt a language, establish a norm, and judge anything outside that context as a deviation from normalcy. This narrow focus restricts our ability to perceive shifts in the landscape and explore new perspectives.

Operating solely for profit does not require brilliance. However, focusing only on profit can place leaders on a path that quickly becomes bleak and insurmountable. It's striking how new businesses face enormous challenges to establish themselves, yet little effort is made to study the main reasons so many fails to thrive.

The paradigms of the world are changing rapidly. While society is creating new forms and values, the world of work remains static, clinging to the old formula of minimizing costs and maximizing revenues to achieve greater financial results and make businesses stand out. This formula has sustained us for a long time because business relationships were once solely consumption-driven, dictated by demand. However, the values driving these relationships are evolving, and new parameters are emerging to balance markets and meet societal expectations.

With every advancement, new relational models arise, reinventing society and creating demands that require reinterpretation and transformation. While I could elaborate extensively on the ongoing changes we face, the truth is that the current shift we're experiencing is yet to fully shape the next wave. Many skeptics argue that this movement lacks strength to drive a revolution, dismissing it as a false prophecy.

However, perspectives will change. Each new cycle leaves less room for doubt while revealing greater dependence on change. This necessitates a shift within individuals, enabling them to find meaning in the emerging business models.

Clients are reexamining their values. Investors are reassessing their priorities. People everywhere are revisiting their principles. There is a clear desire to contribute more to the common good and take greater social responsibility for what they develop in the world. This is not merely about fairer distribution of material wealth but about creating systems that recognize social merit and foster inclusion, enabling each individual to live fully and authentically. This shift is redefining the role of stakeholders and demanding a remodeling of business practices.

Each generation arrives with demands for disruption—not out of a desire to discard the past, but because we ourselves have cultivated new thinking and ideologies. We recognize that value attribution must change. This drives societal innovation, reshaping education, respect for others, and stewardship of the planet. These evolving paradigms demand that we acknowledge the transformative phenomena occurring globally and our role in these changes.

New generations entering the workforce are not impatient because they demand speed for its own sake. Nor are they ambitious because they expect to leap from their first day on the job to the CEO's office in a week. They are not intolerant of longstanding rules and procedures out of disrespect for history. Instead, they have been raised to challenge the status quo, collaborate, make decisions, and execute tasks with simplicity and purpose. If only the CEO's chair offers that opportunity, it's understandable why they aspire to it. By aligning all roles in an organization with the purpose of that chair, we could ease intergenerational workplace conflicts.

We must update our paradigms as quickly as the world evolves. Changes are not driven by machines or nature following its natural course; they arise from people redefining social values and demanding new ways of relating to one another. The workplace and its organizations are integral to this complex entity we call society.

Working solely to achieve profit does not require brilliance. However, focusing only on profit can lead the manager down a path that will quickly prove dark and insurmountable.

For some time, we've resisted change. Yet, the workplace has already transformed significantly since the days of barter and the dawn of capitalism. These past transformations remind us that our current standards and beliefs may also one day be questioned. Future generations may look back and wonder how 21st-century people sustained such controversial, unstable, and punitive work relationships for so long.

During periods of change, understanding and seeing the bigger picture can be challenging. Consequently, we cling to the belief that our positions are correct.

One can imagine someone in 2080 questioning a worker from 2020 about the practices of the time, marveling at the need to congregate in one place, perform repetitive tasks, and endure presence-control mechanisms like fingerprint scans, with punishments for absence, even if the worker contributed significantly to the business. Questions might arise about how special occasions—child birthdays, family deaths—were handled without clear regulations. And what happened if a person wasn't ready to return to work after bereavement leave? The expressions on their faces upon hearing the answers would likely be telling.

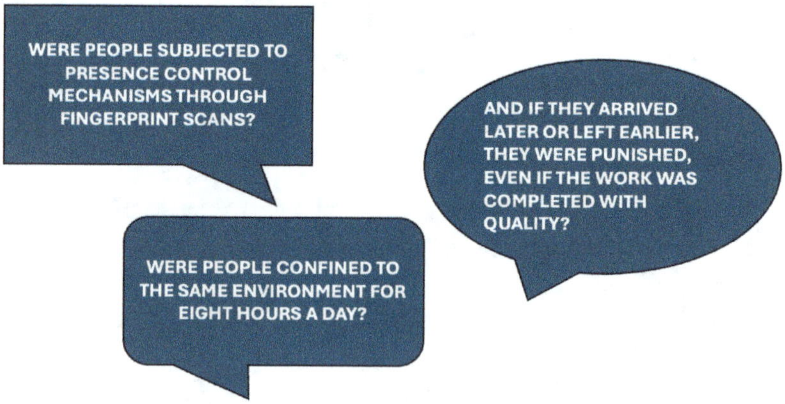

This workplace model is unsustainable. To further damage organizational performance indicators, which fail to create an excellent environment where people can give their best and contribute positively to business success, a similar percentage of managers continue to follow outdated standards without questioning why they do so. These managers impose cost-cutting formulas aimed solely at increasing revenues, failing to realize that low employee engagement leads to exorbitant annual financial losses. Employees deliver less because they cannot tolerate the hostile corporate environments in which they merely survive. It is literally a struggle for survival in the workplace, and this comes at an extraordinary cost to organizations. In the book It's the Manager, Jim Clifton and Jim Harter estimate that, in the United States alone, the annual loss due to low engagement levels amounts to approximately $1 trillion.19

Waking up to the new need for doing business and managing people, as well as breaking down functional barriers where specialists pursue competitiveness and impose their own experiences—segmenting companies into departmental battles—is urgent for recognizing opportunities and fostering collaboration. To begin, I propose shifting the well-known question, "What is the cost of labor?" to "What is the percentage of employees' spontaneous collaboration?"

For example, consider a company where the cost of labor is $1 million, and the collaboration rate is 20% of employees' potential. Compare it to another business with the same focus, a labor cost of $2 million, and an 80% collaboration rate. Which company would achieve higher profitability and productivity?

Entrepreneurship has evolved in appearance and broadened in scope. Previously, society viewed entrepreneurs similarly to investors: individuals who displayed courage and savvy to invest in and own a business. Now, we are witnessing an educational model fostering a new generation of entrepreneurs defined as those who transform the status quo and direct their own destinies, creating innovative ways of doing business in society.

This can manifest through:

- Starting one's own business.
- Associative models, where multiple entrepreneurs combine their strengths to create global change.

- Intrapreneurial actions, innovating within organizations to reshape work processes and foster prosperity and success in corporate settings.

The common thread across all forms of entrepreneurship is society's desire for meaning in all its endeavors. Business creation now inherently connects to purpose and societal contribution. Similarly, participating in existing businesses demands rethinking roles so everyone recognizes the value of their contribution and its alignment with their life's purpose.

These needs are not new but are becoming increasingly urgent, calling for an end to the "modern times" when humans merely keep pace with machines. Competitive models are being questioned, making room for collaborative approaches to social relationships, which also influences the workplace.

Everyone generates greater value when they find meaning in their life's purpose and embrace new, collaborative ways to amplify collective strength. This fosters generosity in doing business and elevates the success of others. A Deloitte study[20] highlights that purpose-driven companies achieve 30% higher innovation levels and 40% greater workforce retention.

Competitors and small supermarket owners in Brazil used to hide their strengths and conceal their weaknesses to avoid being overpowered by the competition. For years, many promising businesses closed because they couldn't compete with large retailers. A group of entrepreneurs saw their fortunes change when they came together and pooled their strengths, creating the Mix Bahia network. Together, they addressed their weaknesses and built a new network, forming an alliance that elevated them to a level of greater competitiveness with large retailers. Combining forces for better purchasing and acquisitions, improved resource management, and enhanced staff training ultimately ensured success for all of them.

The key lesson for investors is that competitors can also participate in the same equation and create a successful model.

New relationship formulas between businesses and customers are emerging, and the paradigms of the past are already

**Each generation arrives with
new demands for disruption,
not simply because they wish
to abandon everything that exists,
but because we ourselves have
fostered new ways of thinking
and new ideologies,
understanding that the way
we assign value must evolve.**

being challenged by the current expectations of the consumer market. **The demand for healthy products, responsible management practices, and conscious consumption is creating impact and meaning in some market sectors,** which are reinventing their formulas in an attempt to reverse significant declines in sales.

Awakening to the new necessity of doing business and managing people, as well as breaking down functional barriers where specialists pursue competitiveness and impose their own experiences – segregating the inner workings of companies into departmental battles – is an urgent step to recognize opportunities and foster collaboration.

Are we obsessed with profit?

Do we recognize our cost-reduction strategies as opportunities for operational performance?

Do we often cut costs in areas that could impact long-term growth?

CHAPTER 7

ELEMENTS FOR CULTURE TRANSFORMATION

Deciphering the Pillars of Engagement (Inspire, Evolve, Care, Thank, and Share)

Imagine five elements that, when combined and moving in parallel, create a harmonious flow of energy, driving changes and transformations in a synchronized way.

Do you know the windmill? Yes, exactly that. A windmill has the perfect mechanism to harness the universe's purest energy—wind—and generate rotations that propel each blade forward. If the blades are colorful, their rapid movement eventually blends into a single, unified color.

One day, at the outset of the transformations we planned to implement at Kordsa—an organization that went through turbulent times in 2010 and 2011 but became an exemplary case of change through people management, recognized as the best company to work for and Company of the Year in 2019 by FIA/Você S/A, and the most incredible workplace in 2020 by FIA/UOL—I sought to understand the foundations that would support the major transformation we aimed to achieve and how we could build an engaging environment.

This led us to identify five key pillars for transformation: **Inspire, Evolve, Care, Thank, and Share**.

The approach was to execute each pillar as part of a cohesive whole, channeling the same level of energy into all five and harvesting the results of this convergence. None were prioritized over the others; rather, everything was to work in unity.

The best symbolic representation of this unified effort was the windmill.

Inspire

After all, how can we inspire so many people and influence their actions toward something greater?

We are talking about the importance of connecting individuals with something bigger than themselves and inspiring them to act with enthusiasm so that each day is better than the last, enabling them to achieve admirable work and align their dreams with everything we are building together.

If a leader cannot articulate where we are going and why we do what we do, it is quite difficult to feel inspired by them. The success of our business must be intimately tied to the ability to fulfill our role within the organization, and this goes beyond recruiting, managing, and concluding the employee lifecycle.

How can inspiration be spread to reach every corner and employee in the company, enabling them to live fully and authentically?

I need to firmly point to our future and speak about it in a way that is simple, clear, and objective so that everyone understands where we are headed. Most people want to experience incredible things in admirable and welcoming environments, knowing what to expect from each team member as they work together to build a story. Knowing where we are going and the challenges each individual will face—challenges that, when combined, will help everyone reach the goal—is a great driver of enthusiasm.

I recognize that in many environments, conversations revolve around goals, and people have no idea where they are going or what those numbers mean. Many do not clearly understand the benefits of what they do daily, yet everyone needs to know where they are headed and how they can contribute.

Slogans like "beating the competition" or "earning more profitability" do not inspire anyone, except those seeking a purely financial relationship with the company. When things start to go poorly, the motivation disappears, and everything tends to collapse.

We must connect people to our dreams. We all know that no one followed the great leaders of history because they shouted, "I have a plan!" Martin Luther King Jr.'s famous statement was, "I have a dream," and in his speeches, he made that dream understandable to his listeners.

Unfortunately, most managers in organizations still proclaim, "I have a plan"—which often hides the full phrase, "I have a plan for you to fulfill my own dream," thereby creating a legion of followers of plans without any personal meaning.

When professionals live their best selves, united by a shared purpose, they connect with the positive impact they have on the ecosystem they are part of, the product they deliver, and the interactions they have with people inside and outside the organization. We believe that anything is possible. If it can be imagined, it can be recognized as already present in the energetic field. We simply need to discover how to connect people to that energy and bring it into the material world.

We can constantly develop new things in pursuit of dreams—or, better yet, **we can develop ourselves through new things when we recognize the transformation this represents for us**.

We have the mission of involving people in challenging goals so they can understand the true importance of what they do, contributing not only to the business but also to their own lives.

The way we communicate must break down barriers, creating accessible dialogue channels and reinforcing trust so that people feel motivated to collaborate with their leaders.

To inspire, it is essential to go beyond organizational walls in search of knowledge, interpreting trends and initiating conversations that allow everyone to recognize we are discussing something greater than what we are today. By exchanging ideas on topics and possibilities that people may not have encountered yet, we help them reflect on how to build bridges from the present to the future.

For senior leadership to acknowledge its role in guiding these dialogues and inspiring the organization, the first question to ask is: "Do we know where we are going?" The next is: "Can I identify what is affecting us right now and the skills we need to develop to address these trends?" Without clear answers, there is no pathway to maintaining organizational engagement. **Trusting the journey and believing we can reach previously unimaginable destinations makes a significant difference for employees**.

It is necessary to understand the role of senior leaders, as well as the leaders who work with people daily. These leaders have an equally crucial responsibility in spreading shared dreams. They need to recognize the challenges their teams will face during transitions and understand that leaders are the primary drivers of enthusiasm.

Most people recognize the importance of two-way dialogue channels, enabling the exchange of ideas and fostering the highest level of contribution across all company levels. However, it is common to find environments where managers do not even invest in one-way communication channels, believing that talking with people is too much work.

If our main role is to lead people so they can live their best experiences and deliver remarkable services and results, inspiring them to make bold decisions and take meaningful actions is the essential pathway to achieving this goal. Guiding everyone in a unified direction is impossible without effective communication platforms.

Engage in regular dialogue with people, whether for specific reasons or not. Have these conversations with employees from different areas of the organization at any time, ensuring you address every individual in every corner of the company without leaving anyone behind.

A High level of engagement and dialogue are proportional in the framework of a high-performance company. The primary factor for achieving high engagement is the frequency of dialogue. In this case, it's not just about informal conversations. People crave formal feedback to understand **where they are headed, what is expected of them, how they are contributing, and how their voices are heard**.

According to research by Great Place to Work, the frequency of feedback correlates with employee satisfaction levels. Employees who receive more than four formal feedback sessions annually tend to have engagement levels above 80%. 21

People want to feel reassured that we trust them, that they can trust us, and that together we can achieve something remarkable to improve the world we live in.
Inspirational individuals are indispensable to a leading company connected with new generations. **Each employee should be inspired to act and think of their work as something far greater than simply performing a task well.** By creating meaning for people, we go beyond inspiration to become passionate about what we do and dream of achieving. We work every day with enthusiasm and seek to expand the vision and impact of every person in our organization.

Connecting purposes keeps people perpetually inspired. By sharing the message of the future and guiding the steps toward transformation, we are continuously challenged to demonstrate coherence and confidence in our teams.

Knowing where we are going and understanding the challenges each person faces—which, when combined, will help everyone reach the goal—is a powerful driver of enthusiasm.

I know leaders who articulate their expectations for professionals to inspire them, invite them to participate in necessary changes, and clearly explain current plans, challenges, and even the losses they face.

Inspiring people is not about pointing out today's losses and how they can reverse them. Business results are not an act of inspiration; they reflect a commitment to performance. Discussions about performance must be conducted with coherence, consistency, and confidence. When results are positive, the dialogue should maintain the same depth as it does during challenging times.

This means upholding principles at all times. If transparency is a core value, it must be preserved in both turbulent and calm periods.

Across all dialogue channels, trust must be the cornerstone. This trust depends on coherence in our communication because people generally know the details. For example, even if frontline employees do not directly know financial performance, this information is readily available to the finance team. Similarly, if sales volumes are satisfactory, be honest, because people are aware.

Such transparency underscores the importance of ethical behavior, as people across the organization know who we are and what we contribute to this broad relationship. If your actions and posture do not align with your words, you are only deceiving yourself and appearing foolish to others.

Every individual deserves respect, including yourself. In summary, you can open multiple dialogue channels, but always ensure coherence and consistency to establish a trusting relationship with your interlocutors.

Strengthen your relationships with everyone you interact with, honor your commitments and promises, and seize every opportunity to expand your understanding through the power of listening.

Before starting a dialogue within the organization, reflect on the importance of being transparent. We often underestimate others' knowledge and treat trivial matters as confidential. However, remember that everyone around you is well-acquainted with your organization. Avoid vague statements, conflicting information, and inaccurate data. If this happens, there may still be inspirational speeches, but people will only join you on your journey if a relationship of trust exists.

After thoroughly considering the significance and commitment of the content you plan to share, I recommend adopting freedom, variety, and creativity. Organize informal gatherings, large team meetings, and focus groups to discuss specific topics that can support your journey alongside your people. Integrate internal dialogue channels with families, society, and everyone you can share your dreams with. Establish avenues for spontaneous suggestions, create internal social networks, set up reporting channels, and implement a code of ethical conduct. **Be as expansive as possible, for the power of leadership dialogue can elevate employees to the highest level of realizing their dreams**.

In parallel with everything we've done, I've always sought to strengthen collaboration with institutions and entities. This approach aims to learn from others' actions and share our practices. By reinforcing the ecosystem and spreading the message of our dreams, we gain support and expand the recognition of our people within society.

Evolve

Evolution walks hand in hand with training. The process of developing and training people is invariably impacted during organizational crises.

First, we must understand what constitutes a crisis versus challenging moments. Some organizations maintain a constant rhetoric of crisis, treating it as their status quo. This requires careful scrutiny of what we broadcast to the world, as true crises often relate to a nation's economic and political landscape. Observing trends in these indicators reveals that while some sectors lament difficulties, others thrive with clear prosperity and stability.

It is true that there are years when economic indicators, such as GDP, show negative results. However, these same indicators more frequently present positive trends. It's worth noting that GDP is an average—if your business shows a negative performance, someone else is experiencing positive results. This calls for an evaluation of your performance, operations, and management

When we set out to discuss performance, we must do so with coherence, consistency, and trust. When results are positive, the dialogue must occur with the same level of depth as it does during challenging times.

**Do you have a clear purpose
and a plan for how you intend
to inspire people
on this journey?**

**Is your intention
genuine and transparent
to everyone?**

**In your dialogues,
are you willing to listen,
share, and be
sincere?**

**Do you believe people
can gradually let go
of distrust and build
a genuine relationship
with you?**

model. One perplexing factor is the tendency to reduce investment in training during challenging times. Development and training are meant to improve performance, enabling people to meet their challenges. Greater training typically leads to higher achievements with fewer errors. Therefore, when someone suggests cutting back on training incentives, I question the logic and long-term outcomes of such decisions. Who is really undermining performance? Who is accountable for decisions that compromise quality? If employees struggle to perform excellently, what is causing this decline?

Another critical aspect is the return on investment (ROI) in training. If investments are made but results are not evident, it likely indicates flaws in the implementation environment or training methods. Halting training, however, does not solve the issue. Instead, the focus should be on intensifying development efforts and improving training practices to ensure returns and expand resources for capacity building. Retaining unqualified personnel is unwise as it can directly harm organizational outcomes.

In times of limited resources, creativity is essential for finding solutions and methods to develop people. Identifying the available talents and optimizing their placement in a structured plan ensures shared learning and growth.

Internal resources alone may not suffice for effective training. When internal expertise falls short, extra effort is required to set priorities and execute necessary training programs. Each investment in knowledge generates multiplied benefits. Thus, turning minimal efforts into significant actions leads to profound organizational transformation.

If the focus lies on existing values and competencies integral to the business, train individuals to transmit this knowledge effectively. Employ methodologies that enhance group learning and extend internal investments, ensuring that everyone strengthens their capabilities.

For boosting performance organization-wide, there are technical approaches that yield direct financial performance improvements, such as process improvement tools, Six Sigma (initially developed by Motorola for optimization), and other quality systems and project management methodologies. These programs deliver measurable financial returns and help monitor resources effectively.

It's essential to recognize that certain skills and knowledge are technical and directly impact employees' ability to perform with diligence. Without investment, task execution suffers, leading to customer dissatisfaction, diminished trust in products or services, and reduced revenue.

The qualifications of your workforce directly influence the quality of products and services delivered to society. Cutting resources without finding alternatives to sustain training undermines the continuity of capacity building.

Establishing a culture of continuous development and learning unleashes the daily potential for human evolution. No interaction between individuals leaves one unchanged—it always offers an opportunity for growth. Each interaction, whether through shared experiences, videos, books, dialogues, or other mediums, creates a natural platform for human development.

The greatest challenge lies in fostering awareness that daily interactions serve as an immense training and development platform. Recognizing these benefits enables us to amplify positive attributes and outcomes within our experiences.

Helping people share their experiences through job rotation programs, practice-sharing initiatives, team project execution, and internal mentorship can yield significant solutions with minimal investment. Strengthening the competency-building profile of leaders and enabling employees to benefit from the expertise of every professional—integrated with the organization's development platform—are just some of the advantages.

If teaching helps us learn, why are we so resistant to creating platforms where our people can exercise their ability to teach?

Internal dialogues, development committees, and providing leaders with the support to act as team developers close the gap between individuals, increase empathy, and foster a knowledge-sharing culture that surpasses any training program.

The organization is a platform for giving and receiving. Helping everyone transform their skills and grow is at the core of human development programs. Companies don't exist solely to profit from work. They first exist to contribute to and shape the society they're part of, enabling growth—and only then do they reap the rewards in the form of excellent work. It is through development that organizations truly thrive.

There can be no organizational development without the awareness, action, and commitment of leaders. We must move away from a model where development professionals are solely responsible for guiding others' growth, transferring this responsibility to leaders. Expanding awareness about the potential for learning, the positive impact on business, and the significance of this process cannot be delegated to other areas of the company. Everyone can assist the leader, but the leader remains primarily responsible for the growth of the people within the organization.

For those with limited resources, it is advisable to engage with associations and professional institutions, exploring development plans through seminars and lectures. These avenues can help distribute resources and create opportunities for professionals to access growth initiatives.

Caring

The act of caring for people goes beyond providing benefits and resources for work. Caring is a gesture of respect, and it helps broaden awareness of what each human being represents within an organization—individuals who dedicate the best of their talents every day to achieve success.

In certain environments, there is not even a minimum level of respect. It's futile to offer numerous resources and benefits if, at their core, people are unhappy and lose the best within themselves—the energy and engagement to contribute.

Providing resources may satisfy people temporarily, but the gains from such a relationship are fleeting. Soon, they return to their state of awareness and evaluate whether the environment is prosperous and whether they feel good in it.

In many workplaces, there are performance metrics to measure management factors such as accident rates, safety, turnover, absenteeism, and more. However, there's one factor that happens daily within companies that would require a gauge for "emotional accidents."

Which talents live their values daily and can help propagate knowledge?

Which specialties within your organization can be structured to be shared with other professionals?

How can personal development be facilitated through dialogue, knowledge transfer, and mentoring processes so that people learn by teaching or learn from those who have experienced it?

Sadly, people may return home physically healthy, protected by measurable performance indicators, yet many carry wounds in their minds or hearts caused by poor-quality interactions with colleagues or leaders who fail to acknowledge the emotional damage inflicted. These issues are invisible to the naked eye, observable only from within, by prioritizing the feelings of the heart. Yet many relationships are so cold, rigid, and abrasive that the harm-doer cannot recognize the damage they've caused.

When engaging with employees, there are always suggestions for improving tools and resources. As trust builds, feedback often includes remarks about leadership styles and the level of respect within the company.

A lack of respect is frequently illustrated by something as simple as the absence of a "good morning" from leaders. While some may dismiss this as trivial, it's worth reflecting on the significance of such greetings. In low-engagement environments, the absence of a genuine "good morning" is common. Even if this concern is deemed unnecessary, consider its deeper meaning.

Social conformity teaches us to greet others. Think back to childhood—your parents insisted you say "good morning," "good afternoon," or "good evening" to everyone in the room. It might have felt torturous, requiring all your courage to mumble a shy greeting while clinging to your parent's clothes. Over time, you were told that these greetings were gestures of politeness and obligation, ingraining the habit.

As adults, many continue saying these greetings, often without making eye contact or with minimal effort, fulfilling what they see as a mere social obligation. In some workplaces, "good morning" is immediately followed by questions like, "Is the report ready?" or "Do we have an update on the project?" This approach can make others feel unimportant.

We rarely pause to consider the essence of these greetings—"good morning," "good afternoon," "good evening." These expressions are genuine wishes for others. If heartfelt, we should deliver them with enthusiasm, truly wishing the recipient an exceptional day—the best day of their life, because it is the present moment.

Reflect on how you greet others. Strive to transform your greetings into genuine wishes. Notice how this small daily gesture alters your relationships with those around you. You'll realize that leadership recognition isn't achieved in a single instance but through consistency and coherence in daily actions.

As adolescents grow into their own, the first thing many lose is the habit of saying "good morning." Sadly, this lapse often starts with those they love most. Genuine greetings are replaced with mundane conversations—complaints about being late, asking if breakfast is ready, pointing out missing items, or discussing daily schedules. We forget to leave our best energy with the people we never want to lose.

It's a simple phenomenon: we lose people day by day. Relationships become mechanical, and we spend a lifetime wondering what went wrong. Often, it isn't a single event but the gradual loss of consistency in expressing care and a lack of awareness about the true meaning of a simple greeting.

This example highlights the fragility of our awareness in relationships. This lack of awareness has turned us into automatic beings, stripping emotions and feelings from our interactions, replacing them with mechanical roles that we perform to perfection. Yet, these roles can compromise our ability to reflect on our actions, leading us to live unmeaningful sequences.

This entire discussion emphasizes that while doing things with simplicity is ideal, **achieving simplicity is far from simple**.

We must genuinely care for our people. The daily reinforcement of the bonds of care and affection that unite us is the source that nourishes us every day. We need to understand our role in the dreams, needs, expectations, and joys of those around us. They expect from us an attitude that is human, approachable, warm, attentive, and friendly.

It's essential to recognize that what drives a company and gives it life are, undoubtedly, the people who work there. **People are the most important element in an organization, and for that reason, I don't refer to them as assets. People come and go, people choose, people persevere, and people quit. They are the engines that give life. Viewing each individual as a complete and unique**

human being is the first step toward treating them with professional respect and personal care. We are complex beings, not mere tools for work, and as such, we have our own expectations and plans.

Caring for people means addressing their essence, feelings, and emotions. It requires understanding that life happens within the organization. **I recommend shifting the concept of "quality of life" to "life of quality." The former promotes a balance between good and bad, while the latter fosters a life that is holistically fulfilling, ensuring quality in all aspects and moments.**

We need to move beyond the rhetoric of valuing effort to genuinely appreciating people for all they contribute.

I've often hesitated to leave work on time in some organizations because commitment was linked to the number of hours worked. This has always been the worst negotiation in history—individuals played the role of the hard worker, but this never truly correlated with commitment. Commitment also includes avoiding unnecessary waste of resources and energy, allowing people to channel their efforts toward achieving the best performance and professional success.

Many leaders demand commitment as if people should act with dedication for no particular reason, doing so voluntarily and with an elevated degree of effort without being asked. However, fostering commitment is very different from the spontaneous dedication that some managers expect in every corner of their organization. Commitment begins with a conscious decision, a desire to do something wholeheartedly, and I've never known anyone to make such a decision without understanding what it entails, its purpose, and the direction it's heading.

For someone to commit, their interest must first be sparked. The object of interest must either generate desire on its own or be presented by someone who demonstrates its importance. Awakening commitment begins with recognizing what matters to the individual, inspiring them, and guiding them toward buying into the idea.

When someone realizes that what they do is connected to their dreams and serves a purpose that can benefit countless others, they open their mind to the idea that their work contributes to something greater. They embrace the idea, take ownership, and develop the desire to do their work every day, becoming agents of transformation themselves.

Consistent and meaningful effort leads to excellence. However, effort without purpose or awareness will not produce excellence or achievement but instead cause pain, suffering, and stress. Caring for people means recognizing that our relationships are not merely professional but also acknowledging that work can aid personal growth and create magical moments in everyday life.

By individualizing our attention, understanding each person as they are, and acknowledging their unique life story, expectations, and beliefs, we can also customize our practices to deliver the greatest possible value to each human being.

A trainee program, for example, can serve as a powerful platform for organizations to nurture young professionals. These programs typically hire students or recent graduates, guiding them through project management and providing a structured learning and experiential environment tailored to their stage in life. Initiatives like these help integrate individuals into the organization, establish mentorship and coaching programs, and create opportunities for rotation to broaden their systemic perspective within the company.

We are complex beings, not mere tools for work, and as such, we carry our own expectations and plans. Caring for people means addressing their essence, feelings, and emotions. Executing these stages with excellence and creating conditions for people to deliver results to their managers, colleagues, and leaders ensures an incredible program.

But there's always room to go further. When we talk about caring, we must consider its importance to the individual. It's about creating a magical, dream-like moment. The concept of **U.D.R.E.A.M.** (Unique, Distinct, Remarkable, Empathetic, Altruistic, Meaningful) is an invaluable tool for ensuring that we address the human element in all our actions. By internalizing this principle and making it part of our daily practices, we can easily ask the right questions to find the best ways to make people truly feel cared for.

How can we help people dream long about our project and forever remember the experience? To achieve this, we must first understand what makes each participant **Unique**. Leaders can ask questions like: “Who is the most important person in this individual’s life?” or “Who would they want to share an unforgettable emotional experience with during their presentation to mark the end of a cycle?” With these answers, we begin to create a singular moment that will be nearly impossible for them to replicate. While the event might include all the standard participants usually involved in company gatherings, we can also invite those who matter most to the stars of the occasion. These could be a parent, an uncle, a grandparent, a friend, or others we might not immediately expect.

This shift from "client focus" to "client-centric focus" is the first step in truly understanding what matters to each team member. While managers may default to naming family as the most important, those who truly know their team understand that meaning goes deeper. Presenting to the most significant person in someone’s life doesn’t exclude others but adds a special value, turning the moment into the realization of a personal dream.

A clear grasp of what is **Distinct** for each individual enables us to break free from repetitive, standardized program formats. It allows each moment to reflect the unique combination of everyone involved. Changing the presentation's location, how people engage in conversations, or the way guests interact can infuse special touches that transform the "how" into something incomparable and unforgettable.

Executing this with excellence brings a sense of **Remarkable** care to the experience. It ensures that every detail resonates with each individual, creating a surge of admiration and leaving a lasting impression.

Making the moment **Empathetic** involves recognizing the energy and spirit required to create a valuable occasion. Such moments must feel fair and meaningful to all involved, ensuring that those experiencing them feel genuinely supported and that their presence is cherished.

The one who crafts the experience becomes a true "magic maker." They do not act out of obligation but from a sincere desire to honor the importance of the other person. Through genuine **Altruism**, they deliver the best possible experience, leaving recipients with the most profound memories, designed specifically to spotlight their protagonism.

Finally, making the moment **Meaningful** is what elevates it from an ordinary compliment or routine feedback to an unforgettable experience. Crafting a magical moment means giving your best to create an experience that the other person wishes could last a lifetime.

The conclusion of a trainee program can often be a repetitive, formulaic event. However, with an innovative design, it can surprise and delight participants by connecting them with those who matter most, allowing them to share their journey and success. This creates an atmosphere of deep connection, linking the trainees, their loved ones, and the organization in a meaningful way.

We sometimes overcomplicate events, investing heavily in resources and protocols while missing the opportunity to forge emotional connections. Speeches by executives and rigid procedures can overshadow what truly matters: evoking emotion as the **foundation of lasting memories**.

We can do things differently! Sometimes, something as simple as providing transportation can create a memorable story by facilitating a connection with loved ones. **Such gestures deepen emotional ties with the organization, solidifying it as the place where individuals have experienced their most cherished professional moment**s.

At times, we focus too much on securing resources to execute our projects, forgetting that most things we need are already available. We have the people we love and a natural desire to connect with them. Yet systems and processes often impose contractual relationships and technical procedures, as if such measures could force or influence behavior.

The lesson is simple: creating meaningful, emotionally resonant experiences doesn't always require grand resources. Often, the magic lies in the genuine effort to understand and honor what truly matters to people.

Connecting with people and the quality of those interactions will determine the quality of the environment we live in. When we feel the need to create procedures and policies to shape professional behavior, it's a sign that we're adhering to flawed standards and beliefs. The higher the quality of relationships, the less we'll need documentation to regulate attitudes and commitments. True commitment stems from embracing something meaningful and relevant to us.

Paying salaries on time isn't a special act; it's an obligation rooted in the employment relationship. Some managers boast about paying market salaries but then expect extraordinary performance. There's a clear inconsistency in this equation. The lack of coherence often lies in the smallest things.

Our journey isn't defined by grand, complex events designed to win people's loyalty or inspire them to connect with organizations. It's the details that are transformative. Consistently and continuously noticing and valuing these details creates meaningful change over time. Such practices prevent us from reverting to the status quo of the past, paving the way for new habits and healthier relationship patterns.

Gratitude

I often hear people increasingly use the term "gratitude," and with each passing day, we express this profound feeling more often. Yet, organizations still undervalue the concept, which is why we need to discuss it.

We see a similar pattern with two other words: reward and recognition. People accomplish extraordinary things in their workplaces and, due to the economic nature of their job, expect financial rewards. Considering that we operate in economic environments generating profitability, it's only fair to share the results with those who contributed. Thus, we all validate this practice.

However, revisiting Maslow's theory, rewards are tied directly to the base of the pyramid, addressing basic needs and enhancing security. The same theory reminds us that social factors are fundamental to our quality of life and are deeply connected to our self-esteem. Therefore, when we achieve something meaningful and noteworthy, it's essential for this achievement to be acknowledged by others, reinforcing personal satisfaction.

This perspective highlights the distinction between reward and recognition. While a reward can be an individual act, recognition requires making the achievement public, allowing the organization to acknowledge the merit.

The first lesson here is that it isn't recognition until the achievement is made public.

You can create various platforms for reward and recognition, such as private or public events. Private acknowledgment demonstrates fairness and values collaboration, yet the sense of happiness and satisfaction it generates is often short-lived.

Public recognition platforms, on the other hand, not only provide momentary happiness but also bring psychosocial factors like group admiration. These effects last longer and, in some cases, remain memorable for a lifetime.

And what about gratitude? Hold on! Hold on! Hold on! Gratitude can accompany both rewards and recognition, yet it also stands alone, independent of either.

Fostering a sense of gratitude in people is transformative, shifting mindsets and personal beliefs, and creating a profound impact in business environments. As I noted at the start, gratitude isn't an action—it's a feeling. It doesn't depend on major accomplishments or outstanding results but rather awakens people to the small, ongoing moments and phenomena shaping their lives every second. It's about recognizing everything that benefits us in some way.

Gratitude broadens our perspective because it's directly tied to acknowledging the elements around us that drive fulfillment. **It reflects on the outcomes of our experiences, considers the positive impact we've had, and expresses appreciation for moments that have advanced our evolution.**

I'm not suggesting a Pollyanna-like view of life, pretending everything is perfect. Instead, it's about recognizing and being grateful for what helps us grow as better human beings. Transformation rarely happens in comfort zones. **Growth stems from confronting challenges, learning from experiences, and adopting new standards for ourselves afterward**.

What are our emotional bonds that foster an excellent work environment?

What are the daily details that strengthen these bonds?

What extraordinary actions can we take to make people feel our genuine care for them?

This evolution isn't about blind acceptance of everything. There are negative actions and situations caused by others that we also need to face and learn from to progress. The question then becomes: How can I achieve a better outcome from this situation than when it started? In the end, **gratitude emerges for having experienced something that set us apart.**

Accepting a situation but staying stagnant, continuing to complain about discomfort without recognizing the opportunity for growth, isn't positive and doesn't contribute to self-improvement. Gratitude doesn't mean clinging to negativity but rather learning and transforming because of it.

Practicing gratitude in an organization involves recognizing that every day we wake up to engage with others. Living in society is as essential as performing tasks and striving for continuous improvement. Every day presents new experiences we've never faced before. Situations will fall out of control, and how we handle them determines whether we grow and evolve.

Again, we encounter the principle of "evolve and serve," magically becoming better through the daily challenges we face. No two days are alike on this growth journey. Therefore, we should show gratitude for every moment and for those who challenge us, as they contribute to our journey.

When we cultivate gratitude, we acknowledge our colleagues' contributions, broaden our awareness of leadership roles, and understand how serving others daily leads to transformative and magical experiences.

We foster gratitude through example, through leaders and collaborators who already appreciate the importance of daily experiences in shaping us as human beings. Gratitude grows through dialogue, which helps us recognize the significance of each challenge, how we handle it, and how we consciously overcome it, enhancing our skills and intellectual toolkit for future adversity.

As leaders, we should always encourage questions like: What did you learn from this experience? What did this moment/situation/dialogue inspire in you that makes you believe you can act better going forward?

People carry immense positive intentions. Everyone teaches in their unique way. When we recognize these differences, we awaken gratitude for everything that elevates us to new heights.

Reward acts are typically based on:

POSITIVE ACTION + TANGIBLE POSITIVE RESULT = REWARD

Recognition acts are generally based on:

POSITIVE ACTION + QUALIFIABLE OR NON-QUALIFIABLE POSITIVE RESULT = RECOGNITION

Gratitude brings a different perspective to everything:

POSITIVE OR NEGATIVE ACTION THAT GENERATED A POSITIVE RESULT = GRATITUDE

Share

When we talk about the importance of sharing with the environment and society, some people may say, "I'd love to, but unfortunately, we don't have the resources to engage in social actions right now."

Sharing goes far beyond financial investment. While the world indeed needs more resources and those who can contribute have a duty to do so, limiting ourselves to the idea of material donations alone undermines the immense potential that a culture of sharing can build within an organization.

We often have something to give, but it isn't always material. We need to break away from the mindset that giving requires material resources and that without them, we can do nothing.

Yes, we are talking about resources, but not all are material. There are two inexhaustible sources of resources we can always share, both of which are invaluable to the world:

Our life experiences—professional, emotional, and educational—can inspire others to adapt our lessons to their own moments and needs, helping them to thrive.

Our attention—offering genuine care, uplifting someone's self-esteem, and finding fulfillment in the act of serving others.

What have you been doing
to foster the feeling of gratitude
in the people who work
alongside you every day?

When you encounter
people who are complaining,
how do you respond,
and what do you ask them
to help them recognize what
they've learned from the situation?

Have you been mindful
in your reward and recognition actions
to ensure that gratitude
is also part of the process?

In addition to these, we can reflect on our daily activities and consider how these processes can serve society by utilizing resources in ways that achieve excellence within a circular economy, where everyone benefits, and waste is minimized. Others can gain from various parts of the process if we include, develop, or redistribute resources effectively.

Inclusion means opening doors to reduce social inequalities, creating opportunities for all, and fostering an organizational culture that serves and uplifts the broader community.

Collaborating with institutions that focus on people's development and social inclusion reshapes internal beliefs and aligns them with society's real needs. By doing so, we can broaden awareness and encourage responsibility for every step of someone's access to our organization. **Recognizing others' challenges cultivates empathy and initiates a journey toward finding effective solutions to close gaps among individuals**.

Establishing diversity and inclusion groups, empowering leaders and volunteers to independently design and execute solutions, strengthens these initiatives, promotes respect, and builds a network of advocates. Regular assessments of these efforts reinforce transparency, deepen organizational awareness, and help evolve mindsets, fostering a culture of empathy and connection to greater causes.

Through this process, refining recruitment, representation, and collective commitment will provide a welcoming environment and achieve better business outcomes. **Diverse thinking generates stronger, more innovative solutions**.

Sharing knowledge, inclusion, and diversity collectively contribute to building an ecosystem where every individual has access to growth opportunities. **The most valuable resource an organization possesses is the ability to share stories of resilience and transformation that involve both the company and its people**.

In every workplace and institution, there are individuals needing support to grow. Inspiring people to share their talents helps elevate others. Many organizations, however, become overly protective of their content, labeling it as "confidential" and thereby preventing the broader sharing of valuable insights with the world.

Sharing success factors creates management models that can improve other organizations and individuals, fostering better businesses, stronger supply chains, and a healthier environment.

For instance, academic partnerships that foster better-trained professionals shorten learning curves once they join your organization. Similarly, better-developed suppliers enhance the quality of your products and services, optimizing performance across the board.

While it's important to protect trade secrets, turning an organization into a mystery stifles opportunities to learn from others and share its strengths with the world.

The concept of a **circular economy** provides immense benefits, including integrating other businesses into our ecosystem. Success is magnified when everyone in the system thrives. Strategic and social partnerships strengthen businesses, reposition their societal role, and create value across entire supply chains.

Organizations that deal with waste daily have opportunities to either find financial solutions or share these materials with others. It's crucial to remember that what we discard doesn't disappear—it simply moves elsewhere and becomes someone else's problem. Imagine if everyone had to carry their own waste wherever they went; we would quickly rethink consumption and reduce unnecessary resources to ensure mobility and sustainability.

Businesses need to open their minds to finding sustainable solutions for the planet to avoid collapse. Integrating processes into their operating environments fosters innovative solutions and creates truly sustainable business models.

Although neglecting circular economy principles may seem advantageous for short-term profits, history teaches us otherwise. Many of the Fortune 250 companies once at the forefront have lost their standing despite their size. As Abraham Lincoln wisely noted, "You can fool all the people some of the time, and some of the people all the time, but you cannot fool all the people all the time."

To build a business that contributes to humanity and leaves a lasting legacy, it's essential to rethink, reposition decisions, and expand the potential to share with others.

Does your secret hinder you from strengthening the ecosystem around you?

How do you share knowledge and the stories of resilience lived by the people in your organization?

How do you integrate into the solutions that your external system and community can offer you?

CHAPTER 8

HUMANIZED LEADERSHIP: THE ENERGY THAT SPREADS AND TRANSFORMS LIVES

Reframing the Art of Leadership

Many people believe that leadership is simply the interaction between a boss and a subordinate, someone in a superior position and someone in an inferior one, as though leadership could be measured solely by hierarchy in a social context. I think this is why organizational structures are so highly valued, as if they define who has the power to lead and who does not.

It is a fact that the art of leadership requires at least two people for the practice of leadership to occur—although it is possible to argue that someone can lead their own life. To be original, I agree that one can lead their own life, but there is much debate about this. Other interpretations of this concept emphasize good planning, discipline, and many other skills that strengthen individuality but do not necessarily impact the life of another person positively.

Thus, we will continue with the magic of leadership through its contribution to enabling another human being to become a better person, with those advancements bringing prosperity to their journey.

Humanized leadership is based on three important pillars, as the act of leading has a much broader impact zone. It encompasses the **ability to build the future, strengthen people's strengths, and develop them for success**.

In this discussion, we will add two other dimensions that must be observed within this principle of humanization. The leadership process should not only focus on personal development—it must go beyond and help the leader to perceive the surroundings and the future of everyone involved, acting in an integrated manner so that the entire ecosystem benefits from their presence.

Some call this a systemic leader because everyone benefits from their actions. Others call them an ontological leader because they act on the essence of human evolution. We will call this type of leadership humanized because our theory, and what we have seen in practice, suggests that humans have gone through evolutionary stages. The first stage was the vegetative and cellular stage—I will not go into detail, as this would lead to a lengthy reflection on the theory of the evolution of species. Following that came our animal stage.

The fact is that we want to affirm ourselves as human beings, yet our habits and behaviors still cause much pain and suffering to those around us, in every environment. There is low tolerance for any behavior or act that contradicts our thoughts and beliefs, and we end up entangled in a sea of physical and psychological violence. In business environments, where happiness, satisfaction, and engagement are low, research consistently shows that people feel they are not treated with respect and admiration.

These factors impose the necessity of promoting humanization in organizational environments, giving purpose to their role in structuring spaces for people's lives. This means creating healthy and welcoming environments that foster the growth of individuals and groups for the betterment of society.

Economic factors must also be considered, establishing integrative, synergistic, and collaborative standards of relationships and collective contributions that favor individual evolution in physical, mental, and spiritual aspects—not addressing religiosity, but the human being's reason for existence and life mission in relation to themselves and their peers.

Leadership is not tied to the power to command, fulfill, and deliver specific results, despite many corporate environments asserting this notion. I want to dispel the myth of leadership based on competitiveness, where the leader is the one who arrives first or occupies a superior position.

We will set aside roles, assignments, and responsibilities, emphasizing that the ability to perform excellent management and ensure the best performance of various organizational resources is indeed an admirable trait in a great leader. However, resource management alone does not determine the quality or level of leadership.

I continue to affirm that leading is not about directing people to perform tasks. Leadership arises from a state of mind whose primary mission is to awaken another human being to live their best every day, fostering their growth, honoring their present moment, and building bridges toward a better future for all.

What matters most to a leader is the other person and everything that leadership can provide to help the other become a better version of themselves, consistently, every day—transforming the small into the great and making every individual extraordinary.

Many people wish to be titled leaders, but leadership is not an act of conquest; it is one of recognition: either others acknowledge you as a leader, or you are not one. People assign this title genuinely, not by imposition, and no organizational role can bestow it.

Only someone who genuinely feels led, who recognizes themselves as benefiting from someone's leadership, who feels supported in their evolutionary process—broadening their worldview and purpose, inspired to seek self-knowledge and self-development daily, and becoming more aware of their personal and professional growth—has the credibility to call someone a leader.

This recognition is desired by many, but few earn it and become the best reference for the development of others.

When someone attains the status of a leader, they undoubtedly embody many positive traits. In a brief exploration of leadership differentiators, particularly for those considered high-potential for the future, three fundamental characteristics stand out, as highlighted by Ram Charan in his book The High-Potential Leader: 22

- Thinking on a Large Scale – Adopting a broad perspective to address challenges.
- Determining What's Needed to Succeed – Securing the tools and strategies required to achieve goals.
- Understanding the Ecosystem – Navigating complexities and fostering collaboration.

From these, countless qualities and competencies emerge—such as trust, systemic vision, and courage. Leaders who leave a positive impact share common traits: they build bridges to the future, promote inclusivity, foster synergy among diverse individuals, and prioritize the development of others.

Leadership is incompatible with those who lack interest in or admiration for humanity, who see time spent developing others as burdensome, and who fail to believe in individuals' potential for growth. Recognizing the value of human beings, their adaptability, creativity, wisdom, and capacity for engagement and harmony is the first step for a leader to earn the coveted recognition.

Business practices often create discomfort when individuals are promoted to hierarchical positions based on technical performance, only to discover they lack the interest or skill to relate to people. This is a primary factor in fostering toxic environments where employees are treated as resources rather than individuals. Many organizations invest in improving their selection processes and accelerating dismissals to offset weaknesses in leadership selection.

Humanized leadership, however, prioritizes cultivating environments where people can thrive, fostering collaboration and mutual respect, and enabling individuals to achieve their best.

Clarity in Building the Future

You have likely heard the metaphor that leaders build bridges.

When leaders focus solely on tasks and factors like quality, speed, efficiency, execution time, and expected results, it can certainly reflect excellent work performance. However, true leadership requires going beyond the immediate scope of the activity. It must reveal to everyone a larger dimension, as leaders hold a broad perspective on the entire context.

How is the engagement level among people in your organization?

What is your process for selecting leaders?

What do the people you've appointed to management roles say about others when speaking (formally or informally) with you?

How are the managers in your organization perceived by the people who work there?

Curiosity is a crucial trait for bridge-building leaders. It drives them to understand the environment around them, recognize trends, identify ways to help individuals in their evolution, and awaken their awareness of the path they are traveling. Leaders aid in laying foundational structures crucial for individuals to develop the tools necessary for future success.

The present is undeniably our best moment because it is the only time we truly have. While the future is fraught with uncertainties, the quality of our present actions, decisions, and steps is directly tied to the inspiration a leader provides. This inspiration broadens our horizons, fosters discovery, and encourages us to craft new solutions to existing challenges. It liberates us, offering peace of mind and clarity to develop our talents and make the most of our journey.

Connection with the future can stir both anxiety and dreams that seem nearly unattainable. Yet, understanding who we are and our potential contributions toward achieving our goals—through conscious steps beyond our comfort zone, embracing change, and focusing on the ultimate purpose of our journey—can bring happiness at every stage. A great leader helps us recognize and value each step along the way.

Powerful questions are those that expand our awareness, making us see possibilities we hadn't previously imagined. **A true leader doesn't impose their vision of the future; instead, they broaden our perspective, enabling us to recognize the future we can create based on our own views, experiences, and life paths.** Each new step must connect with who we are in the present moment, the environment in which we live, and how we can act to transform and create a new reality for ourselves while generating positive impacts for others.

Employees are often trained to provide answers based on the ecosystem's existing framework. However, brilliant and disruptive minds forge new realities by transforming the current state, creating novel scenarios, and rejecting complacency.

To harness this transformative power, we must expand our perspective, broaden our areas of interest, and, more importantly, develop skills in analysis, synthesis, and antithesis. Leaders must question the status quo and help people take steps toward their own evolution.

Expanding the Zone of Awareness and Worldview

For the growth and sustainability of our businesses, it is essential to define and periodically update the map of our organization's impact on the world. By asking questions that awaken our awareness of trends and influences, we activate the necessary indicators to navigate toward prosperity.
Obtaining answers to these questions strengthens our vision and perception of what we contribute, elevating our conscious state. Our success as leaders lies not in having all the answers but in engaging people to reflect and collaborate on constructing new solutions. The collective ownership of finding common answers will solidify our purpose and inspire alignment toward shared goals.

Key Questions for Expanding Consciousness and Driving Business Growth:

The Problem
What is the need our business aims to solve?
What pains exist in the market or the world where our business can make a positive impact?

The Solution
What strengths can we bring to business environments and the world to address these needs positively?

The Intention
What energy drives everything we do, and how does this intention connect with people and systems?

The Benefit
What value do we offer to society, and how does it influence the changes we aim to create and the solutions we want to deliver?

What have you been doing to broaden your worldview?

How do you expand your perspective on everything that positively and negatively impacts your life today?

What questions do you ask to enhance people's awareness?

How do you continually expand your zone of awareness and worldview?

The Uniqueness
What makes us unique in what we do, and how can we strengthen our distinctive value?

The Experience
What experiences do we provide for those who engage with us, and how do they value what we deliver?

The Legacy
Beyond the products and services we offer, what legacy do we leave for the world?

By continually exploring these dimensions, we ensure our organization's alignment with societal needs, enhance its relevance, and establish a meaningful, long-term presence in a constantly evolving world.

Sensitivity to Anticipate Trends

Change will happen, challenges will arise, and often we will be forced to deal with what was not planned.

It is always easier to speak about events after they have passed, as it is much harder to understand the bigger picture and where we are heading while we are in the midst of a particular phase of the journey.

Leaders set themselves apart because they do not follow the motto "let life take me wherever it will." Instead, they are constantly seeking information, observing shifts in scenarios, and, most importantly, connecting with their feelings and emotions to recognize the nuances that transform the reality around them.

It is remarkable how human intelligence can distance us from our instincts, leaving us blind as we cling to the identities we have built and the expertise we have achieved.

Animals retain their instinct to sense trends in their environment, but humans have lost much of this ability, often creating rationalizations to protect their minds and ensure nothing disrupts their satisfaction.

When something good is about to happen, someone important is approaching, or there's a premonition that something negative may occur, animals react early, recognizing these trends as though the energetic field emits advance signals they can detect, allowing them to act based on the accuracy of their instincts. Predators live every day trying to anticipate or disguise these signals to survive, knowing that without cunning, starvation or danger looms.

We observe animals seeking shelter when a storm approaches, taking preventive measures to ensure survival. Humans, however, often disregard such signs, driven by arrogance, believing they are unaffected and superior.

Expanding our perspective to understand trends is not about resistance or paralysis; it is about understanding the context to make the best decisions for the journey we wish to build. It is astonishing how frequently we break relationships, end business deals, or face other changes in life, only to later realize we already knew these outcomes were likely. The problem is that, while we may have sensed them, we often fail to bring this awareness to the forefront to extract the best results and lessons from the experience.

It is unfortunate when we fail even to recognize what happened, missing opportunities to learn and instead repeating the same habits, mistakes, and ways of living.

As leaders, our responsibilities extend beyond ourselves. We know our actions affect others and understand our role in strengthening the foundation for a successful collective journey.

The concept of feeling is much more refined in the leader's journey. While leaders also strive for results like most people, they remain attuned to the signals their bodies and minds present, recognizing the energetic environment they are part of, discerning every hint of change, sensing mood variations, measuring the happiness levels of those around them, and leveraging all these intangible factors to intervene effectively. This ensures they guide others toward the reflections and experiences they need to grow.

If I don't know where I'm going, it doesn't matter what I pack in my bag. Therefore, to recognize the resources we need and how to use them, it's crucial to ask where we are headed and how the winds are blowing in every area, so we are prepared for a successful journey.

Again, I am not dismissing the present but advocating for reading the trends to construct a better future. **Being fully aware of present factors is the best way to envision what lies ahead.** Imagine a navigator embarking on the sea without concern for its conditions, without understanding wind directions, the strength of the clouds, or what is coming. What might happen to this navigator if they simply set sail and let life take its course? It's likely they would attempt to rely on luck and, instead of embracing "let life take me wherever it will," they might end up adhering to "till death do us part."

Political and economic scenarios and business indicators are critical. But they become even more valuable when combined with perception, feelings, and emotions—recognizing people's dreams, learning from challenges, and understanding the unique value every human being brings. This is what fosters brilliance and prosperity.

Creating Solutions Never Before Imagined and Adapted to New Generations

We've already discussed the importance of benchmarking and the challenges it poses for leadership. The world is brimming with ideas, and many have already been tested, making benchmarking a way to shorten the path to successful solutions. However, this resource loses its effectiveness when we blindly copy a model or methodology simply because we admire it, without asking, "Why are we doing this?", "How does this connect with the needs of my organization and its people?", and "What results do we aim to achieve?"

Performance evaluation models were designed and widely disseminated to improve analysis capabilities, aiming to reinforce fair reward and recognition criteria. Quickly, individuals were categorized within distribution curves and quadrants, following recommendations from globally successful models.

Today, many managers strive to foster collaboration within their organizations but fail to understand why people continue exhibiting old, competitive behaviors. Our tools themselves often perpetuate these dynamics, requiring us to reinvent everything we do. Traditional models rarely demonstrate that collaboration is a true value, and in the end, our recognition processes remain rooted in competitiveness. We wish for people to collaborate, yet we continue to glorify the achievement of individual success, leaving others with mere leftovers.

This contradiction is striking, isn't it? We demand creativity and flexibility, advocating for environments where risks are embraced, which inherently leads to more mistakes. However, any deviation from procedures or errors is often met with severe punishment.

At times, it's hard to determine who the rational beings are and who the irrational ones are. Many business decisions and processes lead to minimal success, yet we fall in love with protocols and procedures, prioritizing them over their outcomes or their impact on people's lives.

We must always ask: What are the world's pains? What are the real needs of our customers? And what can we do today to generate the most benefit for those we serve daily?

To create solutions never before imagined, I recommend the following deliberate and sequential steps to boost your innovation potential while eliminating incoherent actions that yield negative outcomes:

Pay Attention: Open your mind to perceive the context and everything around you. Begin by understanding how connections and interferences work and the results they yield. Recognize how current actions influence outcomes. Observe people without judgment—look at their habits, expressions, reactions, sources of inspiration, and exchanges of experiences.

Ask Questions: Question everything within your environment: the practices, actions, and their impact on everyone's lives and results. Assess whether each practice delivers its intended outcomes and gauge confidence levels in these practices. Ask

Are you paying attention to the signals people convey to you daily?

Do you emotionally connect with others and recognize the trends and challenges each individual is experiencing?

Do you have the ability to anticipate risks and competitive advantages by analyzing scenarios?

Do your indicators combine objectivity with subjectivity to inform your decision-making?

whether the tools and methods we use today are admired or just perceived as routine tasks. Identify the complaints and frustrations of employees. Understand the problems they want to solve and organize them to identify congruencies, similarities, and collective concerns affecting many.

Harness Creative Potential: Once you've recognized the needs, involve as many people as possible in generating ideas to address these pains. Present the problems clearly and invite professionals to co-create solutions. Form a "tribe" to stimulate creativity. Use tools like ambient inspiration, brainstorming materials, and creative boards, ensuring contributions are anonymous. Gather as much input as possible.

Plan the Impact: Evaluate each idea within an effort-impact matrix, collaborating with your idea tribe to categorize actions into low effort-high impact, high effort-low impact, high effort-high impact, and low effort-low impact. Prioritize high-impact, low-effort actions first, as they will benefit people the most quickly.

Copying creative processes from others might lead to mismatched applications that clash with your organization's culture. However, be attentive to actions from other areas that could be adapted to meet your needs, forming a new, tailored standard.

Organizations often aim to improve communication processes but struggle with managerial inefficiency in conveying messages effectively. Communication efficiency indicators in low-engagement and low-happiness environments typically mirror poor overall results, making this a significant challenge.

I've encountered business leaders who criticize union representatives for allegedly fostering dissatisfaction. These leaders often adopt hostile behaviors when union representatives engage with employees at workplace entrances. **The first mistake is blaming external forces for internal failures. The second is failing to learn from others' effectiveness.**

Union leaders, for instance, often demonstrate exceptional communication skills, engaging people efficiently where they naturally gather. Meanwhile, many managers resist adopting similar practices, trying instead to enforce rigid communication protocols. This raises the question: Why can't managers communicate directly with employees in those accessible spaces? Why not utilize those channels as well?

Instead of criticizing others' success, leaders should ask questions to uncover the reasons behind their efficiency. By doing so, they can adapt and integrate those talents—possibly already present within their teams—to create innovative solutions that resonate with their unique contexts.

Conflicts among groups and individuals within organizations, even when everyone is striving for the best results for themselves and their teams, often deteriorate collective outcomes. This erosion negatively impacts trust, emotions, and feelings, creating an unpleasant atmosphere that hinders collaboration and damages the collective contribution.

When results falter, and workplace happiness and engagement levels are low, tensions lead to decisions that put people at risk. In a survival instinct, individuals seek ways to protect themselves and avoid negative exposure within the group. This activates the limbic system, causing employees to react defensively to everything and everyone as a means of avoiding vulnerability.

In such scenarios, organizations can turn into battlegrounds. Every time a challenge or issue arises, resistance behaviors emerge, and people deflect attention by pointing fingers at others.

Complementarity in the Art of Leadership

The leader's greatest challenge is to integrate these professionals. However, it's unrealistic to believe that holding a large meeting to announce that everyone must now work as a team and trust one another will lead to instant transformation. Nor can one activity or team-building exercise immediately resolve deep-rooted conflicts.

Once again, the leader's role is crucial. They must act with coherence and consistency to rebuild trust, and this behavior must be reinforced daily to help people reshape their relationships and cooperation.

For this process to succeed, leaders must focus on how they respond to conflicts that arise in daily operations. People, driven by self-preservation, will continue pointing fingers to shift attention and avoid conflict zones. Thus, leaders must address several fundamental points:

Maintain a Holistic View: The problem is always part of a larger context. Leaders must understand how solutions impact the broader ecosystem and influence long-term benefits.

Our minds are often conditioned to focus on problems, neglecting their relationship to the bigger picture. For instance, when someone makes a mistake, we often let that single error overshadow their entire performance, treating it as if it defines 100% of the person. Yet, that error may represent only 0.01% compared to the 99.99% of successes we disregard when emotions run high.

Worse, those around us often amplify the problem, pointing out additional flaws. It's akin to discarding an entire tablecloth because of one ink stain instead of washing it.

Some managers inspect their operations, where people strive daily for excellence, ensuring everything is organized and clean. Yet, when a minor imperfection is spotted, they magnify its importance, devaluing everything else. A better approach would be to help correct the issue collaboratively, demonstrating participation and shared responsibility. This transforms the visit into an act of recognition rather than mere inspection, reinforcing the notion that the team is unified.

Individualize Responsibilities: When problems arise in group settings, it's essential to understand the context and reframe questions. Otherwise, people seeking protection will engage in a blame game, with the most persuasive or well-regarded individuals prevailing in the leader's eyes.

To prevent this, responsibilities must be individualized, and the focus should shift away from criticism toward collaboration. A direct approach is crucial: "I understand that another person is also part of the solution, and I will discuss their responsibilities with them. However, at this moment, I want to know what you can do to help solve the problem and what actions fall under your responsibility."

Political and economic scenarios, as well as business indicators, are very important. But all of this becomes even better when we add a touch of perception, feelings, and emotions, recognizing people's dreams, learning from challenges, and understanding the unique qualities of every individual we encounter. This is what brings us brilliance and prosperity.

This approach discourages deflection and helps address a pervasive organizational issue: gossip.

When people lose the incentive to talk about others and instead focus on their own roles, **conflicts diminish, and communication strengthens. This fosters a collective effort toward common goals, with everyone's responsibilities clearly defined.**

By cultivating a culture of accountability, leaders can transform conflict into collaboration, paving the way for trust and shared success. Effective leadership demands not just addressing challenges but also creating an environment where individuals feel empowered to contribute meaningfully to collective goals.

Identifying Sources of Collaboration and Serving to Prosper

Recognizing strengths to fully utilize available potential is a task that differentiates levels of leadership. But how can we develop leaders to help them identify these strengths?

There are managers who don't even know the names of their team members. If this level of limitation exists, imagine the inability to recognize the strengths of each individual and use them to enhance collaborative potential.

As I have already stated, we are trained to identify vulnerabilities and continue trying to develop competencies in people that are not directly correlated with their talents.

When we create a map of employees to understand their strengths and weaknesses, our management habits often direct us to eliminate weaknesses and shape employees into standard collaborators, within a uniform criterion that we establish as the "ideal model" for the professional profile.

What is your reaction when someone brings arguments about others?

How do you discourage conflicts and gossip in your organization?

How do you ensure the proper assignment of responsibility when problems arise?

How do you avoid being influenced by those who enjoy greater prestige and trust?

Valuing diversity means recognizing that people are different, with different strengths, and that the combination of these advantages can accelerate the process of cooperation, leading to unprecedented results.

The complementarity map can help you identify the strengths of your organization.

STEP 1 - PEOPLE AND TALENTS: Who are the people on our team, and what are their talents?

Learn from each individual about their desires and dreams; the activities they perform in a state of flow, as if nothing else matters; the knowledge they possess and their sources of learning; the skills they have developed over the course of their journey, including those applied outside of the professional environment; and how they respond to various stimuli, demonstrating their attitudes. Understand what these people value and how they express their emotions through what they do and how they do it.

STEP 2 - COMMON GOALS: What does the group truly aim to achieve collectively, and what serves as a motivating factor for them? What do they aspire to accomplish that is fully attainable, and within what timeframe do they intend to achieve it?

Engaging in dialogue with people to identify shared goals enhances synchronicity and helps them recognize they have more in common than they might have thought. Understanding common aspirations and desires facilitates the process of breaking down barriers—often mental ones—that separate individual in different environments. By tearing down these walls, we bring everyone into a shared space of interest and achievement, thereby fostering collaboration and cooperation. We can accomplish more when we realize that, together, we are part of a common and greater objective.

STEP 3 - PERSONAL GOALS: What are the goals of each team member as an individual? Are there personal goals that could potentially be shared to create a common solution?

Leaders differentiate themselves from others because they don't follow the motto "let life take me wherever it goes." Instead, they are constantly seeking information, observing changes in scenarios, and, most importantly, connecting with their feelings and emotions to recognize the nuances that transform the reality around them.

When personal goals have the opportunity to contribute as common objectives for the entire team, we enhance the potential for gratitude and connectivity among individuals. This makes emotional interactions the primary drivers for improving well-being and trust, fostering a sense of community and integrating the workplace as a meaningful part of everyone's lives.

Increasing our individual cooperation levels directly reflects in higher workplace happiness indices, as it strengthens camaraderie and friendship, fostering empathy among colleagues.

STEP 4 - VALUES: Do we know what motivates each individual to get up every day? What principles guide and strengthen them? What are the common values that inspire us to be who we are? What resonates most deeply with the heart of the team?

If we understand the heart as the action of the core, or the action that comes from within, we must recognize the energy that pulses within our team members—what drives them to be who they are, to do what they do, and to sustain the resilience they need when facing adversity. By understanding what matters most to each individual, even for those who may not yet recognize their own values, we foster reflection on the inner strength that can enable them to succeed in who they are and what they do. In this way, we enhance the group's levels of awareness and help its members identify the reasons that sustain their high performance, even in the face of challenges.

STEP 5 - NEEDS AND EXPECTATIONS: What does each team member require to succeed? What are the key needs to increase the chances of success?

We have expectations to achieve our goals, but at times, we lack the appropriate tools for action, which makes the task arduous and difficult. People need to understand which resources will lead them to optimal performance and how to select, facilitate, and implement these resources effectively.

Stating what we want to be done does not compel the universe to deliver the desired outcome. For this, we need the best resources, in addition to understanding that our ability to perform and act with agility is directly tied to the quality and applicability of these tools and our own potentials.

People always want the best resources, and there are moments when it is not possible to meet these expectations. However, we cannot be negligent and demand a high level of performance with a low level of return. This is another factor of learning and awareness that leaders must consider as they broaden their perspective because time, effectiveness, and execution are directly linked to the quality of the tools we have at our disposal.

I know many organizations that provide inadequate resources and demand high performance, but when the expected results are not achieved, they shift the responsibility onto the people.

STEP 6 - ROLES AND RESPONSIBILITIES: What role will each team member assume to ensure success? How will we communicate and keep everyone informed? How will they execute and evaluate the steps completed along the journey?

Leadership is responsible for helping the team understand their roles, with the aim of strengthening cooperation and reducing competition. Clearly defining responsibilities aids in eliminating negative behaviors—such as shifting accountability onto others—and fosters synergy. By focusing their efforts on shared success, team members gain clarity on what the group expects from each individual, develop a comprehensive understanding of the process, and are better equipped to support one another, ensuring that everyone benefits collectively.

STEP 7 - STRENGTHS AND RESOURCES: What strengths do we have as a team that will help us achieve our goals? What interpersonal skills does the team already possess that can be put into practice?

Unlike Step 1, the leader now focuses on embodying the team as a whole, recognizing the behaviors, skills, values, and emotions that, when combined, form the potential collective outcome. At this stage, the group can assess whether the team encompasses all the elements and strengths that diversity provides, including identifying additional assets that may not have been clearly recognized during individual analyses. With all strengths combined, the team can better determine how to implement necessary transformations and how these efforts will benefit the collective.

In this phase, the leader not only becomes more equipped with a comprehensive understanding of the team's talents but also enhances their ability to clarify these strengths, broadening their perspective and contributing to the development of the next generation of leaders.

STEP 8 – WEAKNESSES AND RISKS: What areas does the team need to improve, and what strengths are lacking that must be developed or adopted to enhance success? What should individuals learn about the team and as a team? What obstacles must the team face?

At this point, the reader might be asking: How can one advocate focusing on strengths and then address weaknesses? Indeed, weaknesses are also important; however, our research and decisions do not begin with them. Notice that we never start any process by focusing on individual vulnerabilities. Instead, we first work to consolidate the group, and only then do we identify potential opportunities for development—without trying to mold individuals into a standardized "ideal collaborator" profile.

I prefer to say that all people are the right people; we just need to place them in the exact role where the chemistry of great results can flourish.

We must understand what is missing in the group and what paralyzes it when facing challenges. We aim to identify what makes the team vulnerable and determine what actions can lead to success. In doing so, we acknowledge our weaknesses with the goal of compensating for them by incorporating new talents or developing existing ones.

STEP 9 (OR CENTRAL) - PURPOSE: What is our reason for existing as a team, and how can we bring meaning to everything we do?

Revisiting the construction of purpose may seem unnecessary, but we must recognize that it is both the starting point and the endpoint for consolidating all actions—a guiding force that propels every initiative within an organization.

There's no need for additional questions after the many answers our teams have already discovered. Instead, we acknowledge that the collective engagement of everyone involved enhances the group's commitment to the proposed objectives. A deep understanding of processes underscores the importance of our complementarity, strengthening accountability for each step and organizational need as we grasp what is essential for collective success.

Exercising Positive Influence for the Common Good

We have already highlighted the importance of focusing on the broader context, understanding that any failures or inadequacies that arise are merely opportunities for learning and growth within the larger framework, which far outweighs any single adverse situation.

We must begin with the principle of believing in people, but merely stating this belief is not enough to instill self-confidence and inspire individuals to act creatively in pursuit of the common good.

When we engage with people and express our commitment to their development, **authenticity** in our feelings, comments, and actions is paramount. Words and actions must align.

If we believe that feedback is a vital tool for developing employees, teams, and the organization, we need to demonstrate this belief in practice. There is no better way for leaders to reinforce this concept than by committing to providing five times more positive feedback than constructive feedback.

To differentiate these two formats: Positive feedback highlights actions and behaviors that yield beneficial results and should be recognized every time they occur, accompanied by expressions of gratitude for such performance.

Constructive feedback represents an opportunity to learn, guided by the leader's reflections, which aid in the process of strengthening talents and personal growth.

The goal of delivering more positive feedback isn't solely about its impact on the recipient but also about training the mindset of the one providing it. By seeking out more instances of positive actions, we train our perception to recognize the positive, which in turn influences the environment. A leader who values a positive outlook fosters **well-intentioned**, constructive dialogues, helping individuals become better and establishing a cycle of growth and evolution.

This approach places the leader as **part of the solution**, encouraging team members to identify areas for improvement clearly, reducing the focus on problems and complaints, and fostering genuine personal development.

Maintaining a focus on the positive requires balancing **personalized** and **impersonal** interactions, tailoring conversations to individual profiles, and making everyone feel unique. Leaders must also recognize that people respond to different stimuli and adapt dialogues accordingly. It's crucial to address behaviors, not individuals, avoiding personal judgments and focusing instead on actions where there are opportunities for improvement.

People naturally strive to excel and do their best in every moment. The leader's response to challenges and their approach to addressing them sets the tone for the team's atmosphere and shapes the trust individuals have in being themselves. This trust influences the creation of a positive attitude, enabling everyone to express constructive behaviors when faced with various situations.

Challenges will always arise. The way we respond to them determines whether the environment becomes a source of positive energy or remains stagnant and demotivated due to a lack of confidence.

Unplanned events and adversities are inevitable. Resilience is essential to keep the team persistent and engaged in pursuing collective results. Positive environments enhance the potential for collaboration and drive the achievement of results.

Promoting Synergy

People work together and cooperate on projects when barriers to engagement are removed. However, transitioning from low workplace happiness to high engagement requires additional effort to ensure all participants act with synergy and achieve results collaboratively.

The foundation for assisting people in this journey is creating a work atmosphere where tools and methods for continuous improvement empower them to challenge their beliefs and foster collaborative action through shared projects.

To overcome resistance, it's crucial to start small and pay close attention to details. This approach addresses the need for a mindset shift, reinforcing through the tangible benefits of collaborative work the importance of engaging in activities with shared goals daily.

Continuous improvement programs are well-known in the market. Their primary benefit lies not only in their results but also in their ability to transform beliefs and skills when individuals are challenged to work together. To encourage this, organizations must:

- Select challenging projects to push teams beyond their comfort zones.
- Promote skills and competency training necessary for these projects.
- Ensure consistent support and monitoring throughout each project phase.
- Ultimately, organizations must celebrate together, recognize results, and highlight the positive transformations achieved during the journey.

What have you been doing in situations that threaten good results?

How do you approach people during times of crisis?

How do you help people deal with adversities?

Organizations, depending on their size and resources, can define their continuous improvement strategy by establishing accessible tools. It's essential to ensure employees have the necessary knowledge and support from senior leadership to work confidently, with guidance and encouragement at every stage.

The tools used will depend on the organization's style and culture and how they adapt these resources to their business model. Options include quality training emphasizing principles like PDCA (Plan, Do, Check, Act), Six Sigma, TPM (Total Productive Maintenance), Scrum, Design Sprint, Design Thinking, and other methodologies that align with the organization's resources.

Projects should involve people from different areas and be realistic in scope. Tools and methodologies should match the complexity, difficulty, and scope of each initiative.

Leadership plays a pivotal role in tracking progress. Every leader must act as a supporter and guide, helping define projects, encouraging training, and dedicating time to closely monitor the development of each professional. Leadership's commitment to follow-through and support is what determines whether strategies and execution yield positive outcomes.

This commitment shapes culture. **Managers may set goals and demand results, but leaders develop and guide their teams, enabling them to reach higher levels of personal and professional performance.**

Providing People's Growth

Evolution is inherent to human nature.

Every morning, we wake up and face challenges. By the end of the day, we have evolved through all the situations we've encountered. Interaction between two human beings is necessary for both to acquire new knowledge and insights beyond what they had before the encounter.

People need to awaken to this evolution and become aware of how it occurs. By noticing these transformations, we can better understand and enhance the outcomes of this learning process.

How have you been defining challenges to ensure that people work with a mindset of continuous improvement inherent to the organization's culture?

How do you develop individuals so they acquire the knowledge and skills in key tools that will lead teams to a new level of results?

How do you monitor and support people at every stage of their evolution?

What are clear examples of actions that promote team complementarity?

Engaging in dialogues to help people perceive this evolution is also an important role for a leader. Becoming aware of the changes we experience as we overcome challenges and recognizing the evolutionary process enhances learning potential. It allows us to transition from natural transformation to intentional transformation, enabling us to expand experiences, question our learnings, and analyze how we can improve for future opportunities. This accelerates learning and ensures we face new challenges instead of repeating the same ones.

Every encounter with another person is an opportunity to learn something new. By identifying the quality of these interactions and creating more opportunities for growth, we can systematically accumulate knowledge.

Unfortunately, the habit of judging others hinders our ability to grow from these interactions. When we judge people based on personal preferences like "I like" or "I don't like," we obscure their importance in our growth. We stop asking ourselves about the role this person plays in our life, why they took us out of our comfort zone, and how we can make the most of that situation to learn from the experience.

This is not an argument for tolerating toxic or harmful situations and individuals that hinder our growth and set back our development. In such cases, we must understand what these moments teach us and find ways to prevent harm—moral or psychological. We must remain aware of the thresholds of healthy relationships to avoid crossing from the learning zone into the zone of panic or aggression.

A leader who fosters success helps create an atmosphere of awareness around the evolutionary process, guiding people to complement their essence by understanding their importance in serving better through their actions and creations.

This way, we move from following set tracks, as if life is a predetermined sequence, to navigating trails, using learning to create new moments and experiences, seeking new answers to the same questions, and expanding our worldview.

The practice of learning is liberating and broadens available options. We become new individuals at each stage of development, making it impossible to compare who we are today with who we were yesterday or at any moment in the past. Thus, our present will always be our best version. Understanding this, we take control of our destiny.

Generating Meaning

We must disengage the autopilot and observe transformations. Daily life often feels like a monotonous cycle: waking up, bathing, eating breakfast, brushing teeth, going to work, solving problems, attending meetings, returning home, watching TV, eating dinner, bathing again, brushing teeth, and sleeping—only to wake up and repeat the routine the next day.

If this is the essence of life, we spend years yearning for moments of leisure as a way to break the cycle and find purpose.

Workplaces are transformational and provide experiences that drive growth. Leaders should help individuals understand the nuances of these moments, the significance of each workday, and how to develop themselves for new challenges.

Leadership, at its core, should enable people to become better and optimize how they perform tasks, fostering independence.

The cycle of performance and results requires knowledge of people and the ability to develop vision, talent, and depth as the foundation for any organizational action. **Order** defines processes and execution steps. **Discipline** strengthens competence through the reinforcement of skills and assertiveness in delivering results. **Excellence** should be the ultimate goal to achieve prestige and recognition.

Many personal development models create dependency because they position the company as the provider of resources for growth. After participating in training sessions, employees often expect professional advancement and feel dissatisfied when their contributions are not adequately recognized. This creates a sense of debt in the contractual relationship.

By acting as facilitators in the development process, leaders encourage individuals to reflect on their current growth state and inspire them to pursue opportunities to enhance skills or reinforce strengths.

Knowing individuals—already emphasized in this book—requires no further explanation. Understanding each person's individuality provides leaders with tools to expand dialogue, ask reflective questions, raise awareness, and uncover development opportunities.

Leaders guide the evolutionary process by planning each stage and monitoring self-development to ensure actions are effectively implemented.

Today, multiple sources of knowledge exist, yet people often expect organizations to provide all these resources, reflecting a lack of curiosity and initiative in their own growth process. Leadership must inspire individuals to execute their development plans and ensure, through oversight, that learning genuinely occurs. In this sense, every leader becomes the primary mentor for each person they engage with in the organization, shaping the development process.

In-person training sessions will always hold a special place in the formal perception of learning. However, integrating additional tools into this model—such as coaching by certified professionals or leaders conducting activities and asking questions to help individuals unlock their potential—is crucial. Mentoring or tutoring techniques, using specific tools to accelerate learning, are equally vital. It is also essential to have someone with recognized expertise to guide pathways and enhance technical training. Above all, the leader's role in developing each individual in the workplace remains paramount.

The most significant contribution to professional evolution often comes through project management, assigning responsibilities that challenge the status quo and place individuals in the learning zone, pushing beyond comfort. Guided exploration of successes and mistakes by leaders dedicated to the development process allows employees to become aware of the changes observed in project execution and recognize the significance of each challenge for growth.

The best combination for exceptional performance in people is the union of talent and motivation. Talent must be developed to reach its highest potential as a provider of results when put into practice, but those results will be directly influenced by the level of motivation of the individuals.

TALENT + MOTIVATION = EXCEPTIONAL PERFORMANCE

I often state that no one can give what they do not possess; therefore, our role is to develop people so they can bring out the best of their talents. However, I also frequently repeat another maxim: no one learns what they do not wish to learn.

With these affirmations, we must understand that we need to dedicate our efforts to enabling people to continuously improve their talents so they can deliver their best performance to organizations. Yet, we must remain attentive to the motivation levels of employees, as effort in skill development alone does not guarantee results.

There is a step that precedes the training process: ensuring that beliefs align with leadership expectations. In this case, we need to understand how belief systems operate to dismantle those that are limiting.

Work environments are characterized by their atmosphere, which reflects the collective energy circulating through every space of the organization. It is, in essence, the cumulative representation of all behaviors combined. Aggressive or empathetic reactions to challenges will determine the prevailing environment. By recognizing how these habits interact, we define the culture of the workplace.

The behaviors adopted stem from our competencies or inefficiencies: when competence is high, there is a tendency toward harmony; when deficiencies exist, there is often a tendency to seek protection, which can lead to various types of behavior, including more aggressive ones.

What motivates us to act in one way or another is influenced by our beliefs, which can be empowering or limiting. By delving deeper into understanding people and recognizing the impact of

In every encounter with another human being, we have the opportunity to learn something new. By recognizing the quality of these interactions and providing more opportunities for growth, we can systematically accumulate knowledge.

beliefs on behavior, we can identify what facilitates or hinders the learning process. By using questions that broaden awareness and expand employees' perspectives on the factors blocking improvements in their behavior, we can help them find ways to break free from these limiting beliefs and enter a state of learning flow. This can unlock new resources in their lives, encourage them to adopt new ways of working, and ultimately enhance results and prosperity.

To overcome limiting beliefs, we must help individuals explore the context in which behaviors occur, identify the attitudes generated by these contexts, and understand the consequences of those behaviors. Reflecting on how to break cycles, recognize triggers, and create new behaviors to achieve different outcomes will support professionals in finding better answers and maximizing their potential in their evolution cycles.

Context
The situation in which the behavior was demonstrated.

Expected
The action the person chose to take in response to the situation.

Desired
The impact the action generated as a result.

We have learned that to foster growth, it is essential to help individuals move away from dependency and take ownership of their personal development processes. This involves understanding who they are, recognizing their dreams and desires, evaluating paths that foster conscious evolution through skill development, and awakening their curiosity to explore the many tools available for self-improvement. It also includes expanding their perspective on how workplace development contributes to personal growth and finding ways to enhance this development through projects. Planning with excellence ensures that every opportunity is fully utilized.

Creating Magical Moments

The great challenge for many executives is organizing their time to avoid missing important moments with the people they love. This dilemma is invariably driven by the pursuit of success in their professional careers.

I have been asked how I feel about managing a schedule filled with frequent travel. At the time, my work took me thousands of miles away from my family, and I couldn't spend as much time with my daughters as we might have wished. I calmly responded that the **importance of moments in our lives isn't about their quantity or volume but their intensity and magic**.

The quality of our presence in each moment determines whether we are truly giving it the attention it deserves. Often, we mistakenly believe that spending more time with someone automatically makes it more meaningful. While those who love us may cherish more time together, what they value most is our presence—being genuinely engaged and sharing those moments as if they were unique.

My daughters adore my company, but if I spent every moment with them, considering our generational and interest differences, our relationship might eventually become strained. Imagine an adult constantly hovering over a teenager with no meaningful purpose.

Aggressive or empathetic reactions to challenges will determine the type of environment that will prevail. By recognizing how these habits interact with one another, we define the culture of an environment.

What have you done to increase people's responsibility for their own self-development?

How do you allocate development resources such as research, training materials, coaching, mentoring, and the use of experiences through challenges and projects within their areas of expertise?

What is your level of understanding of each team member's needs and expectations?

When I reflect on my own childhood with my parents, I recall many moments, but the truly unforgettable ones were magical. These memories allow me to relive the emotions, the scents, the flavors, and even the breeze of those times, making them truly unforgettable.

Instead of balancing everything, we need to harmonize our moments. Living in a state of presence means giving the best of ourselves to each occasion and dedicating our best version to those around us, transforming ordinary moments into magical and unforgettable ones.

Humans are capable of multitasking, but the task that truly deserves our full attention should be singular and exclusive. For example, when I'm playing with my youngest daughter, I'm entirely present, giving her the best of me. When I'm at the dinner table with my family, I invest fully in that experience. And when I'm engaging in a dialogue with a team member, I bring my best version to foster a developmental experience that leaves both of us feeling the magic of human connection.

In many workplaces, meetings often provoke negative energy even before they begin. People anticipate them with anxiety, recalling previous unpleasant experiences, and hope the meetings won't take place. During these gatherings, the atmosphere is often expository, aggressive, and focused on stating the obvious, making participants feel like they are merely playing a role. These meetings can feel like a nightmare, with participants wishing the time would pass quickly, as if throwing away minutes of their lives because the time spent wasn't worthwhile. By the end, everyone feels drained.

This might sound tragic, but it's unfortunately common. Blinded by power and unaware of the effects we have on others, we impose unpleasant experiences on people, expecting them to dream of working with us and giving their best every day.

Creating magical moments in the workplace isn't about decorating offices, painting walls, or installing modern recreational equipment. Physical spaces can't make up for negative emotions and reduced contributions from employees.

True magic lies in creating unique, unforgettable experiences for each person we encounter—moments so meaningful that they wish they'd never end. These experiences leave lasting impressions, strengthening emotional bonds and encouraging people to bring their best selves forward, inspired by the positive energy they've received.

You might wonder, what if we're overwhelmed with problems or not achieving results? What can we do when people aren't fulfilling their roles? We can change the way we ask questions, the way we encourage experiences, and the way we foster dialogues.

We can announce a challenge and invite people to seek solutions. We can leverage the group so that everyone can contribute ideas and share their experiences to achieve the desired results. It's an opportunity to focus on identifying the root cause of a problem using logical tools for solution-finding while encouraging team synergy. There are countless things we can do if we adopt a positive outlook toward learning and overcoming obstacles to achieve outcomes that serve the greater good.

I may have a manager who criticizes and pressures, but I can also have a leader who encourages the search for solutions, facilitating the use of tools in a way that helps individuals learn and, over time, overcome their challenges using their own resources and those of others who can assist.

When we talk about someone who leads by example, we promote leaders who seek solutions, demonstrating behaviors that guide their teams toward a higher state of readiness and performance.

Everyone wants to grow and contribute. It is the leader's role to facilitate paths and serve others so that each new moment of learning and experience strengthens the belief that solutions are possible and shapes the mindset to strive for continuous improvement. In this way, people will undoubtedly look forward to meetings, even when the topics are exhausted, because the experience of being there is so enriching that they will want to make the most of the leader's presence.

People who make a difference must also think differently. We need to rethink our habits in executing our roles as managers, understand the magic we can create in corporate environments, and guide people toward a new level of experience.

When we are fully present in the moment, everything else ceases to interfere with the experience, allowing us to be our best selves. Any activity we undertake can be made unforgettable. And since humans shape their conformity through the repetition of patterns, we can set goals to live magical moments more intensely—in family, community, work, and all other areas. Gradually, we will develop healthy habits that harmonize our actions and create positive experiences for those around us.

**At this moment,
only one question remains:
what have you been doing
to create magical moments
for others?**

CHAPTER 9

SERVING TO RECEIVE

We have reached the end of this book, arriving at the fundamental essence of everything discussed so far—the distinguishing factor that separates a leader from a manager. Remember, a leader can be a manager, but being a manager does not necessarily make one a leader. By now, dear reader, you've likely understood the secret.

We hold expectations for people, and within organizations, we desire that everyone be ready to serve and excel in their roles. Look inward and evaluate your role as a leader, living its essence and inspired by your mindset: how much do you serve the people who encounter you daily? How do you create experiences that will drive genuine transformations, enabling them to evolve and serve better?

We already possess all the necessary tools to build a culture of trust and support the development of people, ensuring that the organization thrives with a high level of humanization in its relationships. We recognize both the organizational and individual purposes and know what will lead us to prosperity. However, it is the leader's day-to-day actions—repeated behaviors that demonstrate a genuine interest in fostering the growth of those they lead—that will ensure transformation. This approach guarantees that every experience will contribute to improving our own version of ourselves.

Rather than expecting change from others, we must acknowledge our role and how we fulfill it. A leader first sets the example, instilling confidence in their team to embrace change and develop the new habits they need.

Significant change will come from what we do daily—by expanding our actions and cultivating new supporters until we reach a tipping point where moving forward becomes easier than returning to the old ways. Martin Luther King Jr. built a long journey before delivering his historic speech to 250,000 people in Washington. Steve Jobs had his own path before delivering that unforgettable commencement address at Stanford. These defining moments were preceded by countless smaller actions and speeches that, together, formed a monumental legacy.

When we gain a new level of knowledge and awareness about the factors that shape the world of work and its influence on people's engagement, we also lose our innocence. Continuing to operate from the previous state is detrimental to ourselves and to the society we serve and can help transform.

The art of engagement aims to reduce the emotional "accidents" within organizations, where people show up every day to perform roles devoid of purpose, failing to inspire positive emotions. By helping individuals reframe their careers, these environments can come alive through the quality of relationships and the creation of healthier spaces.

Want to change people's lives? Start by changing your habits. Identify the triggers that sustain your current behaviors and define what you will do to break free from the conformity that yields no results for yourself or others. Strengthen your path to serve, and soon you will see the responses that reinforce your personal transformation for the benefit of the community around you.

The principle of reciprocity will take effect. As you gain your first followers or supporters, nurture those relationships and remain steadfast to build trust and expand your "tribe." Building a tribe committed to doing good and fostering engagement is an act of service to society. Walking alongside your tribe will make it easier to stay calm when faced with critics who dismiss your efforts as fruitless or just a passing trend.

There will be moments when everything seems to be going wrong, and you may feel like giving up. But always remember that we must begin by serving in order to reap rewards in the future. Every change has its optimal performance point. Once you cross that threshold, your mission becomes irreversible, and you will be building a legacy.

START → BELIEVE → CONNECT → TRUST → CHANGE → SHARE → CREATE A LEGACY

Want to change people's lives?
Start by changing your habits.
Recognize the triggers that sustain
your current behavior
and determine
what actions
you will take to break free
from the conformity that produces
no results for yourself or others.

What have you done to fulfill your mission to society through your work?

Who are your loyal followers, and how do you nurture their trust?

What legacy do you want to leave for this world?

REFERENCE

ALMEIDA, E.; KISLANSKY, K. **O poder do propósito**: como viver com mais sentido e potencializar resultados por meio do método Ikigai. Curitiba: Voo, 2019.

BARÉZ-BROWN, C. **Free!**: Love Your Work, Love Your Life. Londres: Penguin Group, 2014.

BUCKINGHAM, M.; CLIFTON, D. O. **Descubra seus pontos fortes**: um programa revolucionário que mostra como desenvolver seus talentos especiais e os das pessoas que você lidera. Rio de Janeiro: Sextante, 2017.

BUSH, M. C. **A great place to work for all**. São Paulo: Primavera Editorial, 2018.

CHAKRAVARTHY, B.; LORANGE, P. **Profit or Growth?** Why You Don't Have to Choose. Londres: Wharton School Publishing, 2007.

CORTELLA, M. S. **Qual é a tua obra?** inquietações propositivas sobre gestão, liderança e ética. Petrópolis: Vozes, 2017.

FERNANDES, M. **Felicidade dá lucro**: lições de um dos líderes empresariais mais admirados do Brasil. São Paulo: Portfolio-Penguin, 2015.

FRANKL, V. **Man's Search for meaning**. Kindle. ed. Beacon Press, 2015.

FREIRE, M. V. **Resolva!** São Paulo: Gente, 2016.

GLADWELL, M. **Outliers**: The Story of Success. New York, Little, Brown and Co., 2008

HALL, K. **Os 4Cs nos negócios**: maneiras rápidas e simples de administrar equipes e projetos nas organizações. São Paulo: Gente, 2009.

HARARI, Y. N. **Sapiens**: A Brief History of Humankind. New York: Harper Perennial, 2015.

RADCLIFFE, S. **Leadership**: Plain and Simple. Londres: FT Press, 2012. SALIM, I.; MALONE, M. S.; GEEST, Y. V. **Organizações exponenciais**: por que elas são 10 vezes melhores, mais rápidas e mais baratas que a sua (e o que fazer a respeito). São Paulo: Alta Books, 2018.

SLIVNIK, A. **O poder da atitude**: como empresas com profissionais extraordinários encantam e transformam clientes em fãs. 8. ed. São Paulo: Gente,
2012.

TRANJAN, R. A. **Não durma no ponto**: o que você precisa saber para chegar lá. 4. ed. São Paulo: Gente, 1999.

NOTES

1 SENA, V. Ranking mostra as áreas com os profissionais mais felizes no Brasil. **Exame**, Dec 1, 2020. Available in: https://exame.com/carreira/ranking-mostra-as-areas-com- os-profissionais-mais-felizes-no-brasil/. Accessed on: May 6, 2022.

2 LEDERMAN, D. Conheça os 7 problemas empresariais mais comuns e como evoluir com cada um. **Lederman Consulting & Education**, 2019. Available in: https://www. ledermanconsulting.com.br/educacao-corporativa/os-7-problemas-mais-comuns-nas- empresas/. Accessed on: Apr 21, 2022.

3 ALLIED MARKET RESEARCH. Global Corporate Training Market to garner $417.21 billion by 2027: AMR. **GlobeNewswire**, Feb 10, 2021. Available in: https://www.globenewswire. com/news-release/2021/02/10/2173383/0/en/Global-Corporate-Training-Market-to- garner-417-21-billion-by-2027-AMR.html. Accessed on: Apr 21, 2022.

4 BARNEY, J. Only 15% of Employees Are Engaged. What Can Leaders Learn? **Einstein Marketer**, 2021. Available in: https://www.einsteinmarketer.com/employee-engagement/. Accessed on: Apr 21, 2022.

5 CRABTREE, S. Worldwide, 13% of Employees Are Engaged at Work. **Gallup News**, Oct 8, 2013. Available in: https://news.gallup.com/poll/165269/worldwide-employees-engaged- work.aspx. Accessed on: Apr 18, 2022.

6 BERMAN, R. Business Apocalypse: Fifty-two Percent of Fortune 500 Companies from the Year 2000 Are Extinct. **Courageous**, 2022. Available in: https://ryanberman.com/ glossary/business-apocalypse/. Accessed on: Apr 21, 2022

7 PEQUENA empresa responde por 70% dos empregos. **Estadão**, Sep 3, 2017. Available in: https://economia.estadao.com.br/noticias/geral,pequena-empresa-responde-por 70-dos-empregos,70001963654. Accessed on: Apr 21, 2022

8 SEGAL, T. Enron Scandal: The Fall of a Wall Street Darling. **Investopedia**, nov 26, 2021. Available in: https://www.investopedia.com/updates/enron-scandal-summary/. Accessed on: Apr 22, 2022.

9 Quanto custa um funcionário desengajado e o turnover alto para a empresa. **Esolidar**, Feb 11, 2020. Available in: https://blog.esolidar.com/2020/02/11/custo-engajamento- de-funcionarios/. Accessed on: Apr 21, 2022.

10 FRANKL, V. E. **Em busca de sentido**: um psicólogo no campo de concentração. Petrópolis: Vozes, 2021.

11 HARTER, J. Managers Account for 70% of Variance in Employee Engagement. **Gallup**, Apr 21, 2015. Available in: https://news.gallup.com/businessjournal/182792/managers- account-variance-employee-engagement.aspx. Accessed on: Apr 21, 2022.

12 OPPONG, T. The inconvenient truths about getting work done. **CNBC**, Jul 10, 2017. Available in: https://www.cnbc.com/2017/07/10/the-inconvenient-truths-about-getting- work-done.html. Accessed on: Apr 21, 2022.

13 A IMPORTÂNCIA de saber ouvir no ambiente de trabalho. **JJ Brasil**. Available in: https://www.jjabrasil.com.br/a-importancia-de-saber-ouvir-em-seu-ambiente-de-trabalho-2/. Accessed on: Apr 21, 2022.

14 5W2H: o que é, como funciona e por que você deveria usar? **Fundação Instituto de Administração**, Feb 11, 2020. Available in: https://fia.com.br/blog/5w2h/. Accessed on: Apr 21, 2022.

15 PAULA, R. Curva de mudança de Kübler-Ross: conheça a 1a teoria de Gestão da Mudança. **VBMC Consultores**, Jan 14, 2022. Available in: https://vbmc.com.br/curva-de-mudanca/. Accessed on: Apr 21, 2022

16 FRANCO, D. **Vidas vazias**. São Paulo: Boa Nova, 2020.

17 JORNADA GPTW: transforme as práticas culturais da sua empresa. **GPTW**, Dec 11, 2020. Available in: https://gptw.com.br/conteudo/artigos/jornada-gptw/. Accessed on: Apr 21, 2022.

18 PATI, C. Conheça as 150 melhores empresas para trabalhar de 2019. **Você RH**, Jan 14, 2021. Available in: https://vocerh.abril.com.br/melhores-empresas/conheca-as-150- melhores-empresas-para-trabalhar-em-2019/. Accessed on: Apr 21, 2022.

19 CLIFTON, J.; HARTER, J. **It's the Manager**: Moving from Boss to Coach. Nova York: Gallup Press, 2019. p. 77.

20 EMPRESAS com propósito têm mais produtividade e crescimento. **Vagas for business**, 2021. Available in: https://forbusiness.vagas.com.br/blog/empresas-com-proposito/. Accessed on: Apr 21, 2022.

21 DINIZ, D. Quanto vale um feedback? **GPTW**, Nov 22, 2016. Available in: https://gptw.com.br/conteudo/artigos/valor-feedback/. Accessed on: Apr 21, 2022.

22 CHARAM, R. **The High-Potential Leader**: How to Grow Fast, Take on New Responsibilities, and Make an Impact. Nova Jersey: John Wiley & Sons, 2017.

ABOUT THE AUTHOR

Luiz França is more than a leader—he is a humanizer of organizations, an inspirer of people, and a catalyst for meaningful transformation. A psychologist with an MBA in Administration and a specialization in people management, Luiz has built a distinguished career across industries such as automotive, finance, mining, paper and pulp, and textiles. As Head of Human Resources and Executive Mentor at EssenceBiz, he challenges outdated paradigms that treat employees as mere resources, advocating instead for leadership that recognizes people as the heart of every organization.

A visionary in humanized leadership, Luiz empowers executives to cultivate cultures of trust, empathy, and innovation. His mission is clear: to help leaders unlock the full potential of their teams by fostering workplaces where people thrive, collaborate authentically, and contribute with passion. His insights have not only shaped high-performing organizations but also inspired professionals worldwide to redefine success—where growth is measured not just by profit but by the well-being of those who build it.

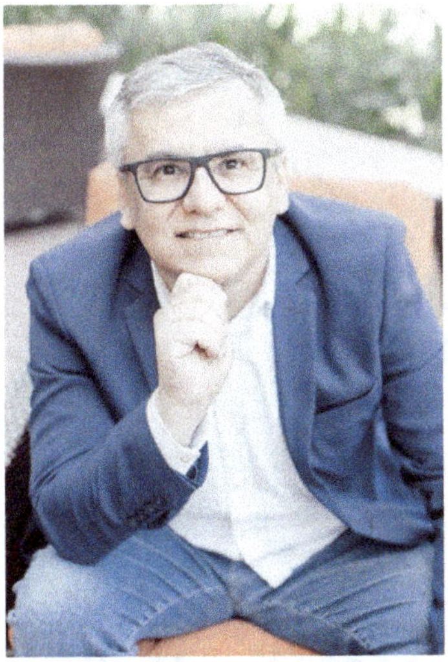

Follow the author in the social media:
INSTAGRAM: LFRANCAOFICIAL
LINKEDIN: LUIZFRANCADUARTE
FACEBOOK: LUIZ-FRANCA
YOUTUBE: LUIZFRANCALF